For Nancy

Michael

July 2004

*Variability
in Human
Drug Response*

True indeed it is, that We do every Day find This to be, in a small Dose, one of the moſt Noble Remedies in the World. But it is not worth the while to engage in the Controverſie warmly debated by ſome *Authors*, how far *Poiſons* are Medicinal; ſince it is notorious enough, that Medicines do ſometimes prove *Poiſonous*. And take the Matter as We pleaſe, it may ſerve to very good Purpoſes to underſtand the manner of Operation of ſo Celebrated a *Drug*, and help Us in a great Meaſure to aſcertain Its Uſe in different Caſes, if we are beforehand rightly appriſed of Its Nature and Way of Acting.

Of opium.
Richard Mead.
In: *A mechanical account of poisons in several essays* (1708).

Variability in Human Drug Response

STEPHEN E. SMITH

MA, BM, BCh, PhD, DA

Reader in Applied Pharmacology and Therapeutics
St. Thomas's Hospital Medical School, London

and

MICHAEL D. RAWLINS

BSc, MD, BS, MRCP(Lond)

Professor of Clinical Pharmacology
University of Newcastle upon Tyne

BUTTERWORTHS

ENGLAND: BUTTERWORTH & CO. (PUBLISHERS) LTD.
                LONDON: 88 Kingsway, WC2B 6AB

AUSTRALIA: BUTTERWORTHS PTY. LTD.
                SYDNEY: 586 Pacific Highway, 2067
                MELBOURNE: 343 Little Collins Street, 3000
                BRISBANE: 240 Queen Street, 4000

CANADA: BUTTERWORTH & CO. (CANADA) LTD.
                TORONTO: 14 Curity Avenue, 374

NEW ZEALAND: BUTTERWORTHS OF NEW ZEALAND LTD.
                WELLINGTON: 26–28 Waring Taylor Street, 1

SOUTH AFRICA: BUTTERWORTH & CO. (SOUTH AFRICA) (PTY.) LTD.
                DURBAN: 152–154 Gale Street

Suggested UDC Number: 615.03

ISBN: 0 407 43300 7

Printed in Great Britain by
Redwood Press Limited
Trowbridge, Wiltshire

Contents

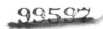

Preface

The aim of this book is to provide practising clinicians and senior medical students with an understanding of why individual patients vary so greatly in their response to drug administration. It is not intended for clinical pharmacologists who specialize in this field; such experts will certainly find much to criticize, in that we have been unwilling to explore in too much depth aspects of the subject which appear to us to be unimportant in the clinical situation or to be poorly understood at the present time.

Much of the book is devoted to pharmacokinetics, an appreciation of which seems to us to be vital if drugs are to be used to their best advantage. Unfortunately, the requisite drug data are scattered widely in the literature, in some instances apparently so widely as to be beyond our ken. Within such limitations, however, we have gathered together the essential information about drugs in current use into a table (Appendix C), which we hope will be helpful to the reader. Much of it was provided by the following pharmaceutical companies to whom we are greatly indebted: Allen and Hanbury Ltd., Astra Chemicals Ltd., Beecham Pharmaceutical Division, Bencard, Boehringer Ingelheim Ltd., The Boots Co. Ltd., Brocades (GB) Ltd., Duphar Laboratories Ltd., Fisons Ltd., Hoechst Pharmaceuticals, ICI Pharmaceuticals Division, Janssen Pharmaceuticals, Kabi Pharmaceuticals Ltd., Lederle Laboratories, Eli Lilly & Co. Ltd., May & Baker Ltd., M.C.P. Pharmaceuticals Ltd., Nicholas Research Institute, Parke-Davis, Pfizer Ltd., Pharmacia (GB) Ltd., Pharmax Ltd., Roche Products Ltd., G.D. Searle & Co. Ltd., E. R. Squibb & Sons Ltd., Upjohn Ltd., Wellcome Research Laboratories, John Wyeth & Brother Ltd. Even so, this table is incomplete and the reader is invited to fill in the missing information as he discovers it. The data provided are the most reliable we could find, but in some

PREFACE

instances we cannot vouch for their accuracy. In particular, some pK_a values derived from different sources disagree markedly; in such cases we have taken whichever appeared to be the most authoritative. We should be glad to learn of our sins of omission and commission.

We thank Elizabeth Rawlins who drew many of the figures. We should like to express our gratitude to the authors and the Editors and publishers who kindly allowed us to reproduce figures and tables from their work; the relevant material is acknowledged briefly and full details are supplied in the references.

We are very grateful especially to Professor G. W. Bisset for his encouragement and criticism during the preparation of the book, and to Professors W. I. Cranston and C. T. Dollery who read through, and Melinda Atthews who typed, the manuscript.

S. E. S.
M. D. R.

CHAPTER 1

Introduction

It is well recognized that the clinical response to drug administration varies widely between individuals. In the case of drugs of small therapeutic ratio (i.e. the toxic dose being close to the therapeutic dose), amounts which prove inactive in some patients can be highly effective and even toxic in others. In some clinical situations such variability can be indicated only in qualitative terms, but in many instances drug actions can be measured quantitatively. In these, variability is expressed either as differing responses to the administration of a defined drug dose or, more precisely, as differing doses required to produce a defined pharmacological action or effect. A few examples serve to illustrate these two modes of expression.

Variability in response to administration of defined drug doses is illustrated in *Figures 1.1, 1.2 and 1.3,* which show frequency distribution histograms of the effects of intramuscular atropine on heart rate *(Figure 1.1),* of phenylephrine eye drops on pupil diameter *(Figure 1.2)* and of oral cyclobarbitone on a test of mental performance *(Figure 1.3).* Variability in dosage required to produce defined effects is illustrated in *Figures 1.4, 1.5 and 1.6,* which show frequency distribution histograms of the anaesthetic dose of intravenous amylobarbitone *(Figure 1.4),* the oral dose of sodium salicylate required to produce toxicity *(Figure 1.5)* and the maintenance dose of oral warfarin required to produce a defined degree of anticoagulation *(Figure 1.6).* Variability in dose requirement of anticoagulant is well known to affect all drugs of the coumarin type (Table 1.1).

The implication of such observations is that in clinical practice the achievement of an optimal response to drug administration requires that dosage be closely matched to the individual patient's requirement. Although such an approach was unimportant at a time when medicaments in common use had only slight pharmacological activity, with the current use of highly sophisticated agents of great therapeutic and toxic potential careful matching is obviously vital. Hence it is necessary to monitor the therapeutic use of anticoagulants and hypoglycaemic

TABLE 1.1. Range of Daily Dose Requirements of Anticoagulants

	Daily dose (mg)	
Drug	Usual	Range
Dicoumarol	75	25–150
Ethyl biscoumacetate	450	150–900
Nicoumalone	4	2–8
Phenindione	100	25–200
Phenprocoumon	3	1.5–6
Warfarin	10	6–25

From Nichol, Keyes, Borg, Coogan, Boehrer, Mullins, Scott, Page, Griffith and Massie, 1958 [3]

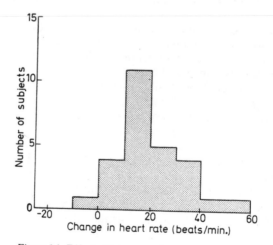

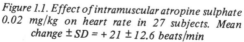

Figure 1.1. Effect of intramuscular atropine sulphate 0.02 mg/kg on heart rate in 27 subjects. Mean change $\pm SD = + 21 \pm 12.6$ beats/min

drugs. It seems likely that great therapeutic benefits would result from the more widespread recognition of the importance of matching appropriate doses to individuals. In this, monitoring of drug therapy, which is discussed in Chapter 10, will inevitably play an increasingly important role. It might reasonably be said that there is at present a greater need for improved methods of using our existing therapeutic armamentarium than there is for the introduction of newer drugs.

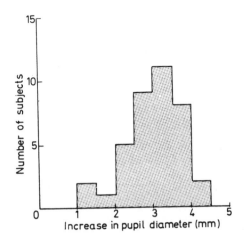

Figure 1.2. Effect of phenylephrine hydro-chloride 30 mg/ml (one drop instilled into the conjunctival sac) on pupil diameter in 39 subjects. Mean change in diameter ± SD = +3.02 ±0.73 mm. (Data from Bertler and Smith, 1971 [1])

From a theoretical standpoint, variability of response of a body tissue to drug administration occurs for two principal reasons: first because different concentrations of the drug may reach the tissue concerned, and secondly because the tissue may respond differently to the particular drug concentration available. In recent years research has improved our understanding of the first of these two aspects of variability; in this book it is discussed in detail in Chapters 2 to 8. Broadly speaking, variability arises because of differences between individuals in rates of drug absorption, in drug distribution and in elimination, either by metabolism or excretion. Although these parameters are discussed separately in this book they are of course related, to the extent that alterations in any one often leads to alterations in the remainder. Thus a change in a drug's distribution inevitably alters its elimination and a change in elimination may alter its distribution. Quantitative aspects of such pharmacokinetic parameters are discussed in Chapter 2. Very much less is known about differences which arise because of variability

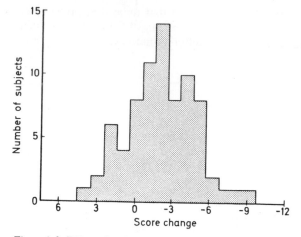

Figure 1.3. Effect of oral cyclobarbitone calcium 360 mg on a test of mental performance (arithmetic ability) in 77 subjects. Mean score change ± SD = −2.0 ± 2.6 columns of figures correctly added. (Data partly from Smith and Sullivan, 1965[5])

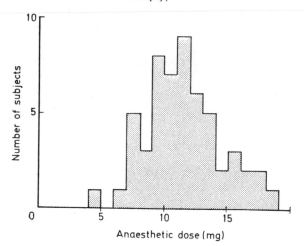

Figure 1.4. Anaesthetic dose of intravenous amylobarbitone sodium in 55 subjects. Mean dose ± SD = 12 ± 2.9 mg/kg. (From Paxson, 1932[4])

in the response of tissues. Studies of responses of animal tissues *in vitro* show remarkable consistency, suggesting that receptors of particular types do not differ noticeably between individuals; and often they are found not to differ even between species. Such investigations are of course performed under highly controlled conditions which cannot be achieved clinically, and it may be unjustifiable to extrapolate such data

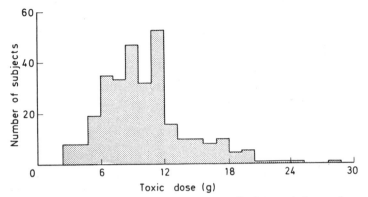

Figure 1.5. Minimal total dose of oral sodium salicylate needed to produce toxic symptoms in 300 subjects. Mean dose ± SD = 10.8 ± 4.0 g. (Data from Hanzlik, 1913[2])

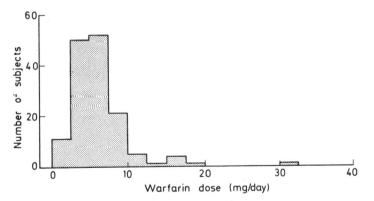

Figure 1.6. Maintenance dose of oral warfarin required to produce anti-coagulation (prothrombin ratio between 2 and 3) among 146 patients under steady-state conditions

to man. Human tissues undoubtedly show interindividual variability in their responses, the differences involved being both quantitative and qualitative. Some of these differences are discussed in Chapter 9.

The presence of disease may alter the effect of drugs or alter dosage requirements in a number of ways. Most obviously, perhaps, in many

5

conditions dosage requirements are related to the severity of the underlying disorder. Such variability is largely predictable and is not discussed here. Disease may also alter absorption, distribution and elimination of drugs with consequent impairment or exaggeration of their effects. Such alterations are discussed in the appropriate chapters which follow. In some situations drug responses may be altered by specific disease influences on the tissues. Hence there is increased susceptibility of individuals with myasthenia gravis to drugs with curare-like actions and of patients with respiratory failure to almost any drug with cerebral depressant activity. Such reactions are beyond the scope of this volume and are not discussed further.

Variability of drug response is also a consequence of a variety of drug interactions which may influence pharmacokinetic parameters, tissue responses or both. Drug interactions are considered in many of the chapters which follow. We do not, however, discuss summation, potentiation or antagonism which arise from straightforward interactions at receptor sites. It is obvious, for example, that coumarin anticoagulants will exert little effect in patients given large amounts of vitamin K_1 and that isoprenaline will have little inotropic influence on patients given beta-adrenoceptor blocking agents. It is equally clear that guanethidine-like drugs will exert greater effects in patients taking diuretics because of summation, or even potentiation, of their hypotensive action, and similarly that alcohol is more likely to induce unconsciousness in patients taking barbiturates. Such interactions are self-evident.

It is apparent from what follows that recent studies have revealed much to account for variability of drug response in the clinical setting. Yet our understanding of this subject is still severely limited because relatively few investigations have been carried out on patients, and in the individual subject it may be difficult if not impossible to deduce why he or she responds in a particular way. Furthermore, experiments on animals do not necessarily yield results which are meaningful to man, often because drugs are given in relatively enormous doses which are well outside the therapeutic range. Even investigations on healthy human volunteers are not necessarily appropriate to the clinical situation, because drugs are often administered in a different form or with greater reliability, or because disease itself often produces disturbances in physiological function which may modify drug action. Many more investigations on patients are urgently needed.

References

1. Bertler, Å. and Smith, S. E. (1971). 'Genetic influences in drug responses of the eye and the heart.' *Clin. Sci.* **40**, 403–410

2. Hanzlik, P. J. (1913). 'A study of the toxicity of the salicylates based on clinical statistics.' *J. Am. med. Ass.* **60**, 957–962

3. Nichol, E. S., Keyes, J. N., Borg, J. F., Coogan, T. J., Boehrer, J. J., Mullins, W. L., Scott, T., Page, R., Griffith, G. C. and Massie, E. (1958). 'Long-term anticoagulant therapy in coronary atherosclerosis.' *Am. Heart J.* **55**, 142–152

4. Paxson, N. F. (1932). 'Obstetrical anesthesia and analgesia with sodium iso-amylethylbarbiturate and nitrous oxide–oxygen: results in obstetrical practice.' *Curr. Res. Anesth. Analg.* **11**, 116–122

5. Smith, S. E. and Sullivan, T. J. (1965). 'The effect of cyclobarbitone on mental performance: a teaching experiment.' *J. med. Educ.* **40**, 294–297

CHAPTER 2

Pharmacokinetics

The term 'pharmacokinetics' was introduced by Dost[7] in 1953 to describe the mathematical analysis of drug quantity and activity within the body. Such an analysis is based on models of the processes of drug absorption, distribution and elimination since it is these which determine drug concentrations within body fluids. The pharmacological activity of a drug depends largely on its concentration at its site of action. Since this is governed by the drug concentration in body fluids, pharmacokinetics is of basic importance in clinical medicine.

Drug absorption

The simplest pharmacokinetic model (Model 1) can be represented thus:

Model 1

Drug in depot   Drug in body   Drug eliminated

$$D_D \longrightarrow D_B \longrightarrow D_E$$

where D_D, D_B, and D_E represent the quantities of drug in the depot, drug in the body and drug eliminated (whether unchanged or as metabolites) respectively. Initially, all the drug administered is represented by D_D, and ultimately by D_E if absorption from the depot is complete. The amount of drug in the body (D_B) at any instant in time is dependent on the fraction of the dose absorbed and the relative rates of the processes of absorption and elimination.

The fraction, F, of the dose absorbed from the depot is represented by:

$$F = \frac{D_{E\infty}}{\text{dose}} \qquad \ldots 1$$

where $D_{E\infty}$ is the amount of drug eventually eliminated either unchanged or as metabolites. F is clearly unity for drugs administered parenterally but is often less than unity for many drugs given orally or rectally. Differences in the fraction of the dose absorbed, whether due to drug formulation, disease or idiosyncrasy, produce considerable differences in the amount of drug in the body at any moment.

In mathematical terms, drug absorption may be considered to occur in one of two ways, as discussed below.

Zero-order absorption kinetics

In the zero-order process, the absorption rate (amount absorbed per unit time, $\frac{dD_D}{dt}$) is constant and independent of the dose. It may be described mathematically as follows:

$$\frac{-dD_D}{dt} = K \qquad \ldots 2$$

where D_D represents the amount of drug in the depot at any time t, and K is the absorption rate with dimensions of amount per unit time (e.g. mg/min). It is described as a zero-order process because strictly speaking the absorption rate is equal to the product of K and the amount of drug in the depot to the power of zero $(D_D{}^0)$, but the latter equals unity $(D_D{}^0 = 1)$.

The simplest example of zero-order absorption kinetics is a continuous intravenous infusion. Constant-rate absorption may also be approximated by various techniques for sustained-release medication. A subcutaneously implanted flat disc, for example, liberates drug into solution at a virtually constant rate from the two opposite surfaces[9] since the area of the edge is negligible by comparison. A subcutaneous or intramuscular depot of any insoluble drug exhibits similar kinetics until the total surface area exposed for solution diminishes significantly. This principle has been used in the design of long-acting ('ultralente') insulins which consist of small zinc insulin crystals of uniform size. Absorption from the gastrointestinal tract may occur by a zero-order process, particularly with sustained-release preparations from which drug dissolution is considerably slower than absorption across the mucosal wall. Dissolution is therefore the rate-limiting step.

First-order (exponential) absorption kinetics

In contrast to the zero-order process, most drugs are absorbed at a diminishing rate $(\dfrac{-dD_D}{dt})$ which is proportional to the amount of drug D_D still in the depot. Thus:

$$\frac{-dD_D}{dt} \propto D_D \qquad \ldots 3$$

and therefore

$$\frac{dD_D}{dt} = -k_{abs}D_D \qquad \ldots 4$$

where k_{abs} is the first-order absorption rate constant with dimensions of reciprocal time (i.e. min^{-1} or $hours^{-1}$). It represents the proportion of drug within the depot absorbed per unit time. The first-order process is so called because the rate of drug absorption is equal to the product of k_{abs} and the amount of drug still in the depot to the power of one $(D_D{}^1 = D_D)$. It is apparent that when first-order absorption occurs the amount of drug in the body reaches a maximum when the absorption rate equals the elimination rate. Thereafter, however, the amount of drug in the body declines. It follows from this that the slower the absorption rate the less is the maximum amount of drug in the body and the less the peak plasma concentration. This is exemplified in *Figure 2.1a* where the predicted plasma concentrations for the same drug, absorbed at different rates, are plotted against time. It can be seen that although the elimination rates and dosages are the same, changing the absorption rate constant from 5.0 $hours^{-1}$ (in curve I) to 1.0 $hours^{-1}$ (in curve II) results in considerably lower plasma concentrations. If the drug were an analgesic requiring a plasma concentration of at least 1 $\mu g/ml$ for a therapeutic effect, a patient in pain with a plasma concentration/time profile resembling curve II would derive little benefit.

Drug elimination

Drug elimination may occur by zero-order or, more usually, by first-order kinetics. In addition, some drugs (e.g. salicylates) are eliminated by simultaneous zero- and first-order processes, whilst others (e.g. phenytoin) are eliminated by apparent zero-order kinetics at higher but

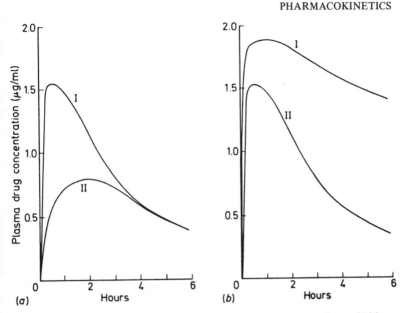

Figure 2.1. Predicted plasma concentrations of a drug given at a dose of 100 mg and distributed with an apparent volume of distribution of 50 l under conditions of differing first-order absorption and elimination kinetics.

(a)   *For curve I, k_{abs} = 5.0 hour^{-1}*   (b)   *For curve I, k_{el} = 0.06 hour^{-1}*
         curve II, k_{abs} = 1.0 hour^{-1}   *curve II, k_{el} = 0.30 hour^{-1}*
     while k_{el} = 0.3 hour^{-1} for both.   *while k_{abs} = 5.0 hour^{-1} for both*

by first-order kinetics at lower plasma levels. For a few drugs the capacity of the enzymes involved in their degradation is limited and at high concentrations the elimination rate approximates to this limiting capacity. For some drugs, therefore, the elimination rate is dose-dependent.

Zero-order elimination kinetics

Under these circumstances, the elimination rate $(-\dfrac{dD_B}{dt})$ is constant. Thus, if D_B is the amount of drug in the body at any time, t,

$$-\frac{dD_B}{dt} = K \qquad \qquad \ldots 5$$

where K is the elimination rate in amount per unit time (e.g. mg/hour). This equation is analogous to equation 2. On integration, equation 5 yields:

$$D_B = D_{B_0} - Kt \qquad \qquad \ldots 6$$

11

where D_{B_0} is the theoretical amount of drug in the body at zero time. For a drug that is completely absorbed, D_{B_0} is the dose. Since, for convenience, it is the plasma concentration which is usually measured and assuming that the drug in plasma is in complete and rapid equilibrium with drug in the rest of the body, equation 6 can be rewritten:

$$C = C_0 - Kt \qquad \ldots 7$$

where C is the plasma concentration at any time, t, and C_0 is the theoretical concentration at zero time. A plot of plasma concentration against time is therefore linear *(Figure 2.2a)*, with slope of $-K$ and intercept on the Y-axis equal to C_0. Examination of equations 6 and 7 shows that the rate of drug elimination *(K)* is independent of both dose and plasma concentration.

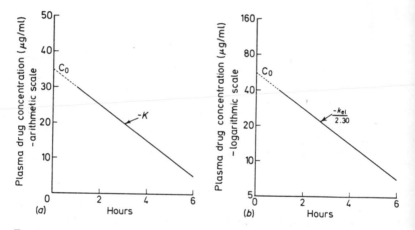

Figure 2.2. Decline of plasma drug concentration with time by: (a) zero-order elimination according to equation 7, where $C_0 = 35$ µg/ml and $K = 5$ µg/ml/hour; the equation fitting this line is therefore $C = 35 - 5t$; (b) first-order elimination according to equation 11, where $C_0 = 70$ µg/ml and $k_{el} = 0.347$ hour^{-1}; the equation fitting this line is therefore $C = 70e^{-0.347t}$

Zero-order elimination kinetics are potentially very hazardous because if the absorption rate exceeds the elimination rate no steady-state is achieved and drug accumulates indefinitely. One example is seen with alcohol[13], the elimination rate of which is constant at about 10 ml/hour. As a consequence, if the intake exceeds this the plasma concentration increases until such time as unconsciousness supervenes!

First-order (exponential) elimination kinetics

For most drugs, the rate of elimination is proportional to the amount of drug in the body (D_B) at any time, t:

$$\frac{-dD_B}{dt} \propto D_B \qquad \qquad \ldots 8$$

and therefore

$$\frac{dD_B}{dt} = -k_{el}D_B \qquad \qquad \ldots 9$$

where k_{el} is the over-all first-order elimination rate constant with dimensions of reciprocal time (i.e. min^{-1} or $hours^{-1}$). This equation is analogous to equation 4. Integration of equation 9 produces:

$$D_B = D_{B_0} . e^{-k_{el}t} \qquad \qquad \ldots 10$$

or

$$C = C_0 . e^{-k_{el}t} \qquad \qquad \ldots 11$$

in terms of plasma concentration (again assuming rapid and complete equilibrium with drug in the rest of the body). It follows that both the elimination rate and the plasma concentration decline exponentially and that therefore a graphic plot of log concentration against time is linear with:

$$slope = \frac{-k_{el}}{\log_e 10} = \frac{-k_{el}}{2.30} \qquad \qquad \ldots 12$$

This is illustrated in *Figure 2.2b*. It can be seen that the time required for the plasma concentration to fall by 50 per cent — the plasma elimination half-life $(T_{1/2})$ — is the same at all plasma levels. Plasma half-life and k_{el} are inversely related thus:

$$T_{1/2} = \frac{0.693}{k_{el}} \qquad \qquad \ldots 13$$

Further detail of the mathematics involved is provided by Riggs[19].

For a drug which is eliminated by only one route, such as the kidney (e.g. benzylpenicillin), k_{el} represents only one constant — the excretion rate constant. Many drugs, however, are eliminated by a combination of metabolism to one or more metabolites and by excretion of unchanged drug. Each process has its own first order rate constant (k_1, k_2, k_3) and

13

the over-all rate constant is the sum of all the individual rate constants for excretion and metabolism thus:

$$k_{el} = k_1 + k_2 + k_3 \text{ etc.} \qquad \ldots 14$$

Rate constants for metabolite excretion do not contribute to the over-all rate elimination constant. Cummings, King and Martin[6] have determined all the individual rate constants for the elimination of para-cetamol, which in man undergoes conjugation with sulphate and with glucuronic acid, only a small fraction being excreted unchanged (*Figure 2.3*). Similar analyses have been applied to the elimination of amphet-amine[4] and nalidixic acid[17].

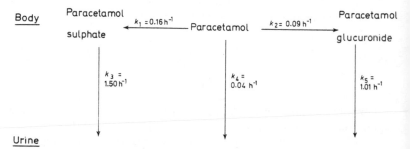

Figure 2.3. Model of paracetamol elimination. The apparent first-order elimination rate constants ($k_1 - k_5$) are shown for each step. Note the slow excretion of paracetamol itself (k_4) into the urine by comparison with its conjugates (k_3 and k_5). The over-all elimination rate constant for paracetamol ($k_{el} = k_1 + k_2 + k_4$) is 0.29 hour^{-1}. (Based on data of Cummings, King and Martin, 1967[6])

Many factors are responsible for variability in the elimination rate of a drug and include sex, genetics, disease and the co-administration of other drugs. These are discussed in greater detail in later chapters. The importance of this variability in elimination rate after a single dose of a drug is illustrated in *Figure 2.1b*, which shows theoretical plasma con-centrations of a drug resulting from the same absorption but two different elimination rates. It is apparent that the therapeutic and toxic effects might differ very considerably in the two situations.

Drug distribution

After a drug reaches the general circulation it is distributed to vari-ous tissues and organs. The rate and pattern of distribution are determined partly by the physicochemical properties of the drug and partly by the anatomical and physiological status of the individual. The total amount of drug in the body and the plasma concentration, C, at any time, are related as follows:

$$D_B = C \cdot V_D \qquad \dots 15$$

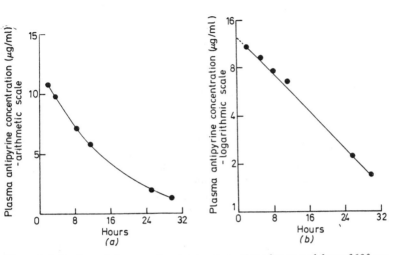

Figure 2.4. Decline of plasma antipyrine concentration after an oral dose of 600 mg at zero time in one subject: (a) arithmetic plot; (b) log_{10} plot. From (b) the following pharmacokinetic parameters can be calculated:

1. *Elimination half-life* $(T_{1/2}) = 10.3$ *hour*

2. *Elimination rate constant* $(k_{el}) = \dfrac{0.693}{10.3}$ *(equation 13)*
    $= 0.0672$ *hour^{-1}*

3. *Theoretical plasma concentration at zero-time* (C_0)
    $= 13$ *$\mu g/ml$ or mg/l*

4. *Apparent distribution volume* $(V_D) = \dfrac{dose}{13}$ *(equation 16)*
    $= 46.2l$

5. *Clearance* $= V_D k_{el}$ *(equation 17)* $= 3.10$ *l/hour*
    $= 51.7$ *ml/min*

where V_D is the apparent volume of distribution. For drugs which are eliminated by first-order processes, the simplest way to determine V_D is to measure the plasma concentration at various times after a single dose. Back extrapolation of the log concentration/time plot (see

15

Figures 2.2b and 2.4) will enable C_0 to be determined, and the apparent volume of distribution then calculated:

$$\frac{\text{dose}}{C_0} = V_D \qquad \qquad \dots 16$$

It is essential that the whole dose be absorbed. In the case of antipyrine *(Figure 2.4)*, which is distributed uniformly throughout the whole body, V_D represents a real volume — the total body water. Most drugs, however, are not distributed uniformly but sequestered in various tissues and bound to proteins. The volume that is measured is therefore an apparent volume and not a real one. This fact is emphasized by reference to nortriptyline which has an apparent volume of distribution in man of 20–50 l/kg body weight[1].

The apparent volume of distribution of a drug is an invaluable pharmacokinetic parameter for two main reasons. First, if the plasma concentration is known, the amount of drug in the body can be calculated from equation 15. Secondly, the apparent volume of distribution can be used to calculate the clearance of the drug:

$$\text{clearance} = V_D \cdot k_{el} = V_D \cdot \frac{0.693}{T_{1/2}} \qquad \dots 17$$

Drug clearance has dimensions of volume per unit time (e.g. ml/min); it is analogous to the more familiar renal clearance but it includes all routes of drug elimination including metabolism. It can be seen from equation 17 that a fall in clearance produces a fall in the elimination rate constant, provided that the volume of distribution remains constant. It is also apparent from this equation, however, that an increase in the distribution volume will result in a reduction of k_{el} if the clearance remains unaltered. It follows, therefore, that changes in the elimination rate of a drug do not necessarily indicate basic changes in drug metabolism or excretion.

Multi-compartmental drug distribution

The foregoing discussion makes the assumption that drug in the plasma is in complete and rapid equilibrium with drug in the tissues and that therefore the plasma contains a constant proportion of all the drug in the body. Under such circumstances the drug is distributed as in a single compartment. Such an assumption is invalid if the drug penetrates relatively slowly into, or emerges slowly from, tissues of large capacity. In these conditions pharmacokinetic analysis of the drug's distribution requires a more complex model containing two or more body compartments. The simplest such model (Model 2) can be represented thus:

Model 2

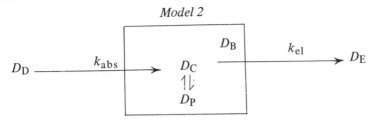

In Model 2, D_D, D_B and D_E represent the quantities of drug in the depot, drug in the body and drug eliminated, as before. However, drug in the body is divided into two compartments, a central compartment (D_C) and a peripheral one (D_P), between which drug exchange occurs relatively slowly. Differences between D_C and D_P may be determined by differences in tissue perfusion or by sequestration of the drug in tissue depots or by protein binding.

Drug elimination from a multi-compartmental system does not obey first-order kinetics but follows a multi-exponential decline. Thus, from a two-compartment system the decline is bi-exponential (i.e. the sum of two exponentials) as illustrated in *Figure 2.5*. From a three-compartment system elimination is tri-exponential, and so on. Constants for two-compartment models can be calculated[14, 18, 19] and the methods have been applied to the kinetics of lignocaine[20], chloroquine[11], nortriptyline[1], reserpine[12] and amylobarbitone[3]. A three-compartment system[10] has been used to describe the plasma decline of dicoumarol following intravenous administration[15].

To the extent that tissue perfusion, sequestration and protein binding are themselves complex, it might be thought appropriate to construct more complicated models still to match particular plasma concentration/time profiles. Four-, five- or six-compartment models could be devised in theory but in practice their individual characteristics would be indistinguishable. Under such circumstances, when drug elimination follows a multi-exponential decline, an approximation to the observed decline may be given by the equation of a power function:

$$C = A \cdot t^{-\alpha} \cdot e^{-\beta t} \qquad \ldots 18$$

where A, α and β are constants[2]. Such an equation describes the decline in plasma levels of buthalitone *(Figure 2.6)* in man more closely than does the more conventional three-compartment analysis[22].

17

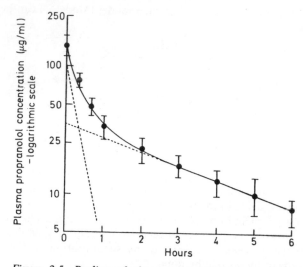

Figure 2.5. Decline of plasma propranolol concentrations (mean ± SD) following intravenous administration of propranolol 10 mg to five subjects. The bi-exponential decline (dotted lines) on this log concentration/time plot indicates distribution of the drug according to a two-compartment system. (From Shand, Nuckolls and Oates, 1970[21])

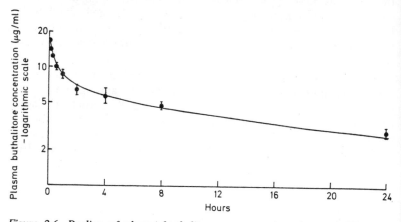

Figure 2.6. Decline of plasma buthalitone concentrations (mean ± SE) in 19 subjects following intravenous administration of buthalitone sodium 11 mg/kg. The line is calculated according to the power function $C = A.t.^{-\alpha}.e^{-\beta t}$ (equation 18) where $A = 23.9$ μg/ml; $\alpha = 0.252 \times 10^t$ (min); $\beta = 8.427 \times 10^{-5} t$ min. (After Smith, 1972[22])

The importance of ascribing the correct model to pharmaco-kinetic studies is twofold. First, it allows more accurate determinations of the apparent distribution volumes and elimination rate constants. Secondly, it allows concentration/time profiles to be constructed for the particular compartment in which the drug exerts its pharmacological effects.

Multiple-dose kinetics

The preceding account has been confined almost exclusively to the pharmacokinetics of single-dose drug administration. In clinical practice, however, the majority of drugs are given with a multiple-dose regimen. The relationship between the mean steady-state plasma concentration (C_{ss}) and the various pharmacokinetic parameters described earlier is given by the following equation[24]:

$$C_{ss} = \frac{F \cdot \text{dose}}{V_D \cdot k_{el} \cdot T} \qquad \ldots 19$$

where T is the dosage interval in time. Examination of this equation shows that the steady-state plasma level during multiple dosing is directly related to the dose and the fraction of the dose absorbed (F), but in contrast to the plasma concentration after a single dose (see above) it is not dependent on the absorption rate. Equation 19 also demonstrates that the steady-state plasma level is inversely related *both* to the apparent volume of distribution and to the first-order elimination constant (i.e. the plasma clearance). The dose and the dosage interval are (nominally) under the control of the prescriber but the fraction of the dose absorbed, the elimination rate constant and the apparent volume of distribution are all characteristics of the individual patient. Intra- and interindividual differences in any of these pharmacokinetic parameters result in differences in the steady-state plasma level. Of these parameters, k_{el} appears to be the major source of variability although the contributions of V_D and F are by no means negligible. *Figure 2.7* shows the predicted plasma concentrations of the same drug at two different elimination rates when given at fixed, repeated intervals and at the same doses. Curve I (with the smaller k_{el}) attains a higher steady-state plasma concentration than curve II, and takes longer to reach steady-state conditions. It has been shown on a theoretical basis[23] that when a drug is given at a fixed dosage at constant intervals, 90 per cent of the steady-state plasma level is reached after 3.3 elimination half-lives; about 5 half-lives are required to reach steady-state. Too frequent increases in dosage for drugs with long half-lives may result in excessive cumulation and possible toxicity; this can take several days to develop.

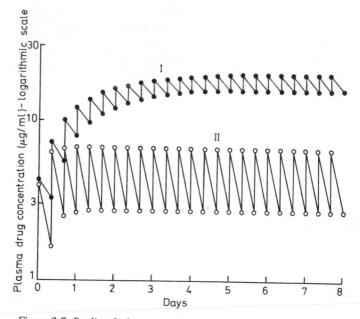

Figure 2.7. Predicted plasma concentrations of a drug given at a dose of 200 mg 8-hourly for 8 days. The distribution volume (V_D) is the same (100 l) for both curves but the half-life is 24 hours in I and 6 hours in II. Note in I the higher steady-state concentration and the longer time required to reach it

Kinetics of pharmacological effects

It has been assumed in the preceding discussion that there is a relationship between the amount of drug in the body (or plasma concentration) and its pharmacological effect. Without this relationship the foregoing account would bear little relevance to clinical medicine.

The increasing effect of most drugs with increasing dosage is well known. This can be regarded as indicating that the greater the amount of drug in the body the greater is the effect. After single-dose administration of a drug which equilibrates rapidly between the plasma and its 'receptor compartment' (i.e. its site of action), it should be possible to demonstrate a good correlation between plasma level and effect, provided that the drug acts reversibly and that its metabolites are inactive. Such appears to be the case with pentazocine[5] *(Figure 2.8)*. The situation becomes more complicated, with a drug such as warfarin, which produces its maximum reduction in prothrombin activity after about 2 days, when the plasma level has diminished to below half its maximum value. However, by relating the logarithm of the plasma

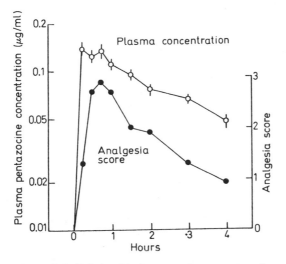

Figure 2.8. Relationship between plasma pentazocine concentration (mean ± SE) and analgesic effect after a single intramuscular dose of 0.64 mg/kg to eight subjects. (From Berkowitz, Asling, Shnider and Way, 1969[5])

concentration to the clotting factor synthesis rate at any time it is possible to demonstrate a clear linear relationship[16] *(Figure 2.9).*

Although few workers have attempted to correlate pharmacological effects with plasma drug concentrations after single doses, even fewer have explored correlations of such effects with steady-state plasma concentrations during multiple-dose regimens. One exception is the elegant study by Freyschuss, Sjöqvist and Tuck[8] which explored the relationship between nortriptyline administration and its effect of reducing the pressor response to intravenous tyramine. As shown in *Figure 2.10,* the reduction in tyramine sensitivity was highly correlated to the steady-state plasma nortriptyline concentration ($r = 0.81$) but unrelated to the daily drug dose ($r = 0.18$). The importance of the pharmacokinetic variability found is clear.

It is not to be expected that all drugs should show a relationship between plasma level and pharmacological effect. Thus drug metabolites may contribute to such effects or the effects may be modified by

21

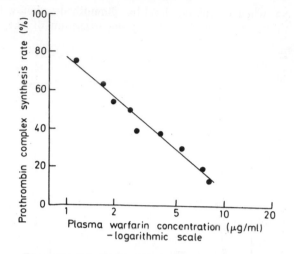

Figure 2.9. Relationship between prothrombin complex synthesis rate and plasma warfarin concentration under different dosage conditions. (From Nagashima, O'Reilly and Levy, 1969[16])

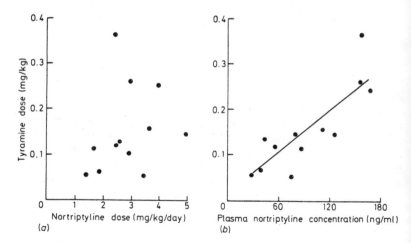

Figure 2.10. (a) Lack of correlation between tyramine pressor response (dose of tyramine required to produce a 20 mm Hg rise in systolic blood pressure) and nortriptyline dose (mg/kg per day) in 12 individuals under steady-state conditions. (b) Correlation between tyramine pressor response and steady-state plasma nortriptyline concentration (ng/ml) in the same individuals. (From Freyschuss, Sjöqvist and Tuck, 1970[8])

22

homoeostatic processes or tachyphylaxis. Furthermore, disease or inter-individual differences may result in altered tissue response. Such influences are discussed in Chapter 9.

References

1. Alexanderson, B. (1972). 'Pharmacokinetics of nortriptyline in man after single and multiple oral doses: the predictability of steady-state plasma concentration from single-dose plasma-level data.' *Eur. J. clin. Pharmac.* **4**, 82–91
2. Anderson, J., Tomlinson, R. W. S., Osborn, S. B. and Wise, M. E. (1967). 'Radiocalcium turnover in man.' *Lancet* **1**, 930–934
3. Balasubramaniam, K., Lucas, S. B., Mawer, G. E. and Simons, P. J. (1970). 'The kinetics of amylobarbitone metabolism in healthy men and women.' *Br. J. Pharmac.* **39**, 564–572
4. Beckett, A. H. and Tucker, G. T. (1968). 'Application of the analogue computer to pharmacokinetic and biopharmaceutical studies with amphetamine-type compounds.' *J. Pharm. Pharmac.* **20**, 174–193
5. Berkowitz, B. A., Asling, J. H., Shnider, S. M. and Way, E. L. (1969). 'Relationship of pentazocine plasma levels to pharmacological activity in man.' *Clin. Pharmac. Ther.* **10**, 320–328
6. Cummings, A. J., King, M. L. and Martin, B. K. (1967). 'A kinetic study of drug elimination: the excretion of paracetamol and its metabolites in man.' *Br. J. Pharmac.* **29**, 150–157
7. Dost, F. H. (1953). *Der Blutspiegel: Kinetik der Konzentrationsabläufe in der Kreislauffüssigkeit.* Leipzig: Thieme
8. Freyschuss, U., Sjöqvist, F. and Tuck, D. (1970). 'Tyramine pressor effects in man before and during treatment with nortriptyline or ECT: correlation between plasma level and effect of nortriptyline.' *Pharmacologia Clin.* **2**, 72–78
9. Goldstein, A., Aronow, L. and Kalman, S. M. (1968). *Principles of Drug Action.* New York: Hoeber; London: Harper & Row
10. Loo, T. L., Tanner, B. B., Householder, G. E. and Shepard, B. J. (1968). 'Some pharmacokinetic aspects of 5-(dimethyltriazeno)-imidazole-4-carboxamide in the dog.' *J. pharm. Sci.* **57**, 2126–2131
11. McChesney, E. W., Fasco, M. J. and Banks, W. F. (1967). 'The metabolism of chloroquine in man during and after repeated oral dosage.' *J. Pharmac. exp. Ther.* **158**, 323–331
12. Maas, A. R., Jenkins, B., Shen, Y. and Tannenbaum, P. (1969). 'Studies on absorption, excretion and metabolism of ^{3}H-reserpine in man.' *Clin. Pharmac. Ther.* **10**, 366–371
13. Marshall, E. K. and Fritz, W. F. (1953). 'The metabolism of ethyl alcohol.' *J. Pharmac. exp. Ther.* **109**, 431–443

14. Martin, B. K. (1965). 'Kinetics of elimination of drugs possessing high affinity for the plasma proteins.' *Nature, Lond.* **207**, 959–960

15. Nagashima, R., Levy, G. and O'Reilly, R. A. (1968). 'Comparative pharmacokinetics of coumarin anticoagulants. IV. Application of a three-compartment model to the analysis of the dose-dependent kinetics of bishydroxycoumarin elimination.' *J. pharm. Sci.* **57**, 1888–1895

16. Nagashima, R., O'Reilly, R. A. and Levy, G. (1969). 'Kinetics of pharmacologic effects in man: the anticoagulant action of warfarin.' *Clin. Pharmac. Ther.* **10**, 22–35

17. Portmann, G. A., McChesney, E. W., Stander, H. and Moore, W. E. (1966). 'Pharmacokinetic model for nalidixic acid in man. II. Parameters for absorption, metabolism, and elimination.' *J. pharm. Sci.* **55**, 72–78

18. Riegelman, S., Loo, J. C. J. and Rowland, M. (1968). 'Shortcomings in pharmacokinetic analysis by conceiving the body to exhibit properties of a single compartment.' *J. pharm. Sci.* **57**, 117–123

19. Riggs, D. S. (1963). *The Mathematical Approach to Physiological Problems.* Baltimore, Md: Williams & Wilkins

20. Rowland, M., Thomson, P. D., Guichard, A. and Melmon, K. L. (1971). 'Disposition kinetics of lidocaine in normal subjects.' *Ann. N.Y. Acad. Sci.* **179**, 383–398

21. Shand, D. G., Nuckolls, E. M. and Oates, J. A. (1970). 'Plasma propranolol levels in adults with four observations in children.' *Clin. Pharmac. Ther.* **11**, 112–119

22. Smith, S. E. (1972). 'General pharmacological principles.' In *A Practice of Anaesthesia*, p. 938. Ed. by W. D. Wylie and H. C. Churchill-Davidson. London: Lloyd-Luke

23. Van Rossum, J. M. (1968). 'Pharmacokinetics of accumulation.' *J. pharm. Sci.* **57**, 2162–2164

24. Wagner, J. G., Northam, J. I., Alway, C. D. and Carpenter, O. S. (1965). 'Blood levels of drug at the equilibrium state after multiple dosing.' *Nature, Lond.* **207**, 1301–1302

CHAPTER 3

Drug Absorption

When a drug is given by any route except intravascular, the time of onset, the duration and the intensity of its action are determined partly by the characteristics of absorption from the site of administration. This chapter is concerned exclusively with absorption from the gastrointestinal tract, not because variability in absorption from other sites is unimportant but because its determinants are largely predictable from knowledge of the physical state of the drug and the existing local circulation at the site of administration. It has long been known, for example, that absorption of insulin from subcutaneous sites is determined by the physical state of the preparation (viz: soluble, amorphous or microcrystalline), and that depot preparations of benzylpenicillin and corticotrophin are absorbed more slowly than their soluble counterparts. Similarly, the addition of adrenaline to solutions of local anaesthetic agents prolongs their local effects by retarding absorption into the general circulation. Factors which influence inhalational, percutaneous, enteral and parenteral drug absorption are well discussed in published reviews[7, 12, 25, 61].

From the gastrointestinal tract absorption is possible anywhere from the mouth to the anal canal, although when drug preparations are swallowed (as the majority are) most absorption occurs from the small intestine largely because of the enormous mucosal surface area and blood supply available there. Absorption of most drugs occurs by simple diffusion across the lipoprotein cell membranes of the intestinal mucosa. Lipid-soluble forms are therefore most readily absorbed. In the case of weak electrolytes, which exist in ionized and non-ionized states, only the latter are lipid-soluble and consequently available. Absorption is therefore critically dependent on the extent to which the drug is in the non-ionized state at the pH of its surroundings. This in turn depends on its pK_a or ionization constant (the pH at which it is 50 per

25

cent ionized), values of which are given in Appendix C. Absorption of weakly acidic drugs such as salicylates and phenylbutazone occurs partly from the stomach because these drugs are largely in the non-ionized state at the pH of the gastric contents.

Although drug absorption clearly varies greatly between individuals the reasons for this variability are not always obvious. In a study of absorption of guanethidine in a small group of hypertensives, McMartin and Simpson[44] showed that some subjects absorbed as little as 3 per cent and others as much as 27 per cent of the administered dose. This difference may well contribute to the known extreme variability in dose requirement (from 10 mg to 1,000 mg/day) for the management of hypertension[49]. A number of contributory factors could be involved in such a clinical situation:

(1)   reliability or unreliability of drug taking;
(2)   drug formulation;
(3)   pH of the gastric contents;
(4)   presence of food and other substances in the lumen;
(5)   gastrointestinal motility;
(6)   intestinal absorptive function.

These factors will be discussed separately, though it is important to realize that in many instances failure of drug absorption may occur for a variety of these reasons in combination. Indeed, in many clinical instances the precise reasons may not be known. Furthermore, we discuss here factors which influence the passage of drugs from the gastro-intestinal lumen into the portal circulation, whence such drugs pass to the liver. During this first passage, significant quantities of drug may be inactivated by intestinal and liver metabolism, variability of which inevitably contributes to the apparent variability of absorption into the systemic circulation. This is discussed in Chapter 5.

Reliability or unreliability of drug taking

It comes as something of a surprise to many doctors that patients do not always take prescribed drugs. Even among hospital in-patients drug consumption may not be absolutely reliable, especially if the prescriptions involved are complex and multiple[60], even though dispensing of drugs from ward stocks is monitored carefully. Among out-patients and in general practice unreliability of consumption is both a common cause of treatment failure and a saving grace where drugs with marked side-effects are concerned.

Much attention has been drawn to unreliability of consumption of iron tablets in pregnancy, a finding which is usually ascribed to the occurrence of unwanted gastrointestinal symptoms. Doubt must be cast on this interpretation, however, since Kerr and Davidson[33] found an equal incidence of such symptoms among subjects receiving iron and lactose and since out-patients are known to exchange unpleasant symptomatology among themselves[14]. Two investigations under trial conditions have indicated an average consumption of iron tablets of about two-thirds of that prescribed[10, 51], but it seems probable that among patients under routine antenatal care consumption is much less. This is unfortunate because failure to take iron tablets in pregnancy often contributes to iron-deficiency anaemia[10].

Serious consequences also attend unreliable consumption of oral antibiotics for the treatment of bacterial infection. Mohler, Wallin and Dreyfus[47] found that about two-thirds of their patients with streptococcal infection took the full one-week course of penicillin prescribed but the remainder took less, usually because they felt well, not because they misunderstood the instructions. Even more depressing figures have been reported[5] among children for whom a ten-day course of oral penicillin was prescribed for pharyngeal infection. By the third day of the course 56 per cent and by the sixth day 71 per cent had stopped treatment, as assessed by tablet counts, liquid preparation measurements and in most instances by urinary antibiotic assays. In every case the parents said that the treatment was given exactly as instructed. On long-term chemotherapy for tuberculosis spot testing of urine for para-aminosalicylate (PAS) has also revealed substantial patient unreliability[18, 41], which is presumably due to the occurrence of side-effects.

Defaulting on the taking of prescribed drugs has also been shown in the treatment of depression with imipramine[51]. It seems likely that compliance with instructions is poor among patients on most tricyclic antidepressants and the major phenothiazine tranquillizers because of the frequency with which these drugs produce unwanted side-effects. In a careful study of patient co-operation in a trial of antirheumatic drugs, which also frequently produce side-effects, Joyce[31] has shown how measures of reliability of tablet taking and patient co-operation can be used to improve the sensitivity of a clinical trial of drug treatment. Social and demographic comparisons of reliable and unreliable tablet takers have shown no clear differences[6]. Medication error is the subject of a recent review[55].

Drug formulation

The availability of an active drug in an oral preparation for absorption from the gastrointestinal tract has long been the concern of pharmaceutical manufacturers, and the idea that some preparations may be better in this respect than others is not new. The subject has, however, received much publicity in recent years because of findings

TABLE 3.1. Contents of a Typical Sugar-coated Table for Oral Administration

Constituent	Content (mg)
Tablet core	
ABC 789 (active substance)	5.0
Dimethyl silicone oil	0.5
Polyethylene glycol 6000	0.5
Benzensulphonic acid	2.05
Polyvinylpyrrolidone	3.0
Sucrose	3.0
Talc	3.0
Maize starch	6.0
Lactose	26.95
Coating mass	
Indigotine pigment	0.171
Cetyl alcohol	0.017
Arachis oil hydrogenated	0.017
Stearic acid	0.104
Polyethylene glycol 6000	0.104
Silicic acid	0.174
Polyvinylpyrrolidone	0.174
Cellulose	0.304
Titanium dioxide	0.869
Talc	1.035
Sucrose	7.031
Total tablet weight	60.000

From Freestone, 1969[22]

that marketed preparations differ widely, often with serious consequences. In most countries these marketed products fulfil requirements of pharmaceutical authorities (such as the British Pharmacopoeia and the United States Pharmacopeia) which usually stipulate that tablets and capsules must have a drug content which falls within certain limits (e.g. ± 10 per cent) either side of the advocated content and that they must disintegrate *in vitro* within a specified time. However, limits on particle size within the preparation, dissolution times of the active principle and the nature and quantity of excipients present are rarely dictated. Contents of a typical sugar-coated tablet, including diluents, binding agents, lubricants for manufacture, disintegrating agents and dyes are indicated in Table 3.1. Such diversity of content offers plenty of scope for variability in disintegration, particle size and dissolution. The result is that although most products fulfil pharmacopoeial standards the availability of drug to the patient is exceedingly variable. This has been termed 'generic inequivalence'[59] and the availability of the drug for absorption 'bioavailability'.

Differences in bioavailability have been reported for many drugs. The most important must be for those which are very expensive, are rather poorly absorbed or require close dosage control. Obviously the last-named is the most critical. Particle size was found to be of major importance in determining bioavailability of spironolactone, absorption increasing about tenfold from microparticle preparations[4]. This observation enabled a preparation ten times more potent to be marketed commercially. More recently, a similar change has influenced marketing of digoxin, following several reports of differing bioavailability among preparations of different manufacturers. The most astounding of these reported sevenfold differences in peak plasma concentrations following administration of different preparations in single doses[40]. Lesser, but significant, differences were found in other studies[45, 54]. In all these instances the limiting factor was probably the rate of dissolution of the drug, which has been shown to differ widely[46]. *In vitro* characteristics of the 'old' and 'new' commercial digoxin tablets produced by one manufacturer are illustrated in *Figure 3.1.*

Variable absorption is critical also with the oral hypoglycaemic agent, tolbutamide. Varley[59] compared a commercial and a pharmacopoeial preparation in respect of absorption and blood glucose response and found them to differ three- to fourfold in bioavailability (*Figure 3.2*). The importance to the diabetic patient of maintaining supplies of the same bioavailability is obvious. A change in tablet make-up was responsible for an outbreak of phenytoin toxicity among epileptics in Australia. Tyrer and his colleagues[58] reported an association between toxicity and the use of lactose instead of calcium sulphate as excipient. Toxicity disappeared when the manufacturer reverted to the original formula. The reason why the calcium salt reduces phenytoin bioavailability is not known, but it might act by altering disintegration and dissolution characteristics. Dissolution rates have also

29

been found to vary among different preparations of warfarin although, interestingly enough, without resultant differences in bioavailability[63]. Apparently absorption of warfarin, though possibly

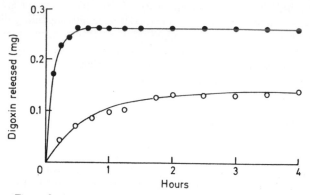

Figure 3.1. Dissolution profiles of two preparations of digoxin in vitro. (From Fraser, Leach and Poston, 1972[21])

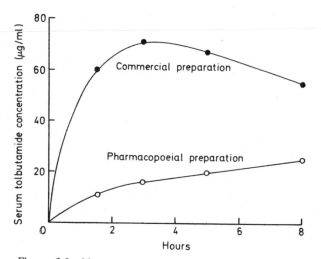

Figure 3.2. Mean serum tolbutamide concentrations (10 subjects) following oral administration of tolbutamide 1 g as a commercial branded preparation and a pharmacopoeial preparation. Ratio of areas under the lines = 3.57. (From Varley, 1968[59])

delayed by slow dissolution, remains complete so that total bioavailability is unimpaired. The observations illustrate the need to distinguish between *rates of absorption* which might be expected to influence clinical efficacy of drugs requiring high peak concentrations (e.g. in chemotherapy and when they are used once only) for reasons discussed in Chapter 2 and *totality of absorption* which should influence drugs of slower action and turnover as well.

Antibiotics are subject to bioavailability problems. Thus peak plasma levels and total urinary excretion of chloramphenicol have been found to vary some three- to fourfold between preparations[24]. Similar, though less marked, differences can also affect tetracyclines[3, 8, 11], prednisone[13], triamterene and hydrochlorothiazide[57] and a number of analgesic drugs such as phenylbutazone[53], paracetamol[28] and indoxole[62]. Absorption of salicylates is greatly influenced by the solubility of the drug itself, the rate increasing with increasing solubility. Thus aspirin, buffered aspirin and sodium aspirin, as shown in *Figure 3.3*, are absorbed at quite different rates[37], though whether these differences affect total absorption or therapeutic

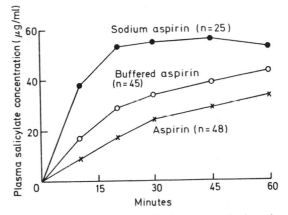

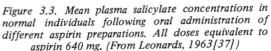

Figure 3.3. Mean plasma salicylate concentrations in normal individuals following oral administration of different aspirin preparations. All doses equivalent to aspirin 640 mg. (From Leonards, 1963[37])

efficacy is not known. Specially designed dissolution tests have been shown to predict quite accurately aspirin absorption rates in man[38]. Buffering and solubilization of aspirin preparations is also associated with reduced likelihood of gastric bleeding, probably because increased ionization reduces lipid solubility and consequent absorption into gastric mucosal cells. There have, however, been reports of patients with rheumatoid arthritis and gastrointestinal lesions who have bled after taking buffered aspirin preparations.

pH of the gastric contents

Absorption of weakly acidic drugs through the gastric mucosa is impaired if the gastric pH is greater than normal, either because of achlorhydria or as a result of antacid consumption[12]. Although in theory this might reduce the efficacy of a wide variety of drugs including antipyretic analgesics, anticoagulants, barbiturates and hypoglycaemic agents, the influence is only slight probably because most absorption occurs from the small bowel even though the pH conditions there are less appropriate. One exception appears to be carbenoxolone, absorption of which is completely inhibited by a rise of gastric pH above 2 [20]. This drug must therefore not be taken at the same time as antacid compounds such as aluminium hydroxide and magnesium hydroxide or trisilicate, or it will not be absorbed locally into the cells on which it acts by promoting mucus production[26], nor have its expected beneficial effect on gastric ulcer healing. An advisable regimen would be to take the carbenoxolone before the meal and the antacid after it. Neglect of this precaution may account for some therapeutic failures with the drug.

Antacids also inhibit absorption of tetracycline antibiotics, although the effect has been ascribed not to an alteration of gastric acidity but to chelation of the metal ions of the antacid by the drug. Thus calcium, magnesium, iron and aluminium salts all have the same effect[35]. Sodium bicarbonate reduces total absorption of tetracycline from commercially available capsules but has no effect on absorption of solutions of the drug[2]. The likely explanation is that sodium bicarbonate, or perhaps the increase in gastric pH, inhibits dissolution of the capsule. It remains to be seen whether the other metal salts mentioned have the same action.

Gastric contents are known to empty more rapidly into the duodenum when the intragastric pH is raised. On a theoretical basis, therefore, intestinal absorption ought to be accelerated by the consumption of antacids. This may be responsible in part for the increase in availability of drugs like salicylates when they are consumed in alkalinized preparations (see discussion above and *Figure 3.3*).

Presence of food and other substances in the lumen

Drug absorption is delayed by the presence of food in the stomach. Thus the consumption of antibiotics after a meal leads to lower blood concentrations than when the drugs are taken on an empty stomach. This could clearly render such treatment ineffective if the plasma and tissue concentrations are reduced too far. Serum concentrations of cloxacillin and cumulative urinary excretion of sulphadimidine following administration of these drugs in fasting and postprandial subjects are shown in *Figures 3.4 and 3.5*. In each case delay in absorption is apparent. Similar findings have been reported for most penicillins[42, 56] and more recently for paracetamol[43]. The clinical significance of these findings is clear; for best effect, drugs should be taken on an empty stomach whenever feasible.

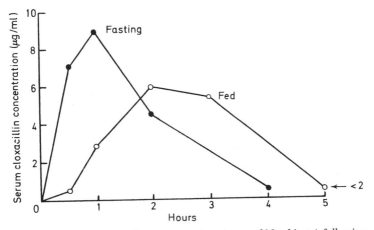

Figure 3.4. Serum cloxacillin concentrations (mean of 10 subjects) following oral administration of cloxacillin 500 mg fasting or fed. Areas under curves are the same. (Data from Knudsen, Brown and Rolinson, 1962[34])

Of less obvious influence is the presence of chemical substances and even certain foods in the lumen of the intestine which have a specific effect on absorption. Thus eggs have been reported to reduce iron absorption[36] and a high intake of fat aids absorption of griseofulvin[16].

Substances which interfere with the absorption of fat and of fat-soluble vitamins such as liquid paraffin and cholestyramine may also influence drug action. Chronic consumption of these agents can lead to relative deficiency of vitamin K and thus could theoretically potentiate the coumarin type of anticoagulant such as warfarin and phenindione. However, recent work has indicated that cholestyramine has the opposite effect in practice because it binds the anticoagulant in the gut lumen, thus reducing the amount available for absorption[29, 52], just as *in vitro* it can bind these and a number of other similarly acidic agents[23]. The adsorptive properties of activated charcoal recommend

33

this substance for clinical use in the treatment of acute aspirin poisoning for similar reasons[17, 39], although the charcoal must be given soon after the aspirin. It is obvious, however, that casual consumption of charcoal tablets or biscuits by patients may have the undesirable effect of reducing the absorption and thus the effectiveness of drugs deliberately prescribed for treatment.

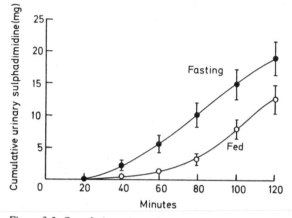

Figure 3.5. Cumulative urinary free sulphonamide excretion (mean ± SE) following oral administration of sulphadimidine 0.5 g fasting (20 subjects) or following rice meal (20 subjects)

Interactions between drugs can also influence absorption, although the mechanisms involved are obscure. Chymotrypsin administration has been reported to enhance blood levels of phenethicillin[1], presumably by increasing absorption and possibly by reducing binding to proteins in the intestinal lumen. By contrast, a barbiturate (heptabarbitone) has been reported to inhibit absorption of dicoumarol, with consequent reduction of its hypoprothrombinaemic effect[48]. This finding is of considerable interest because barbiturate-induced tolerance to anticoagulants of this type is usually assumed to be due to enzyme induction and increased metabolic inactivation (see Chapter 7). Clearly other factors may be involved as well. Defective absorption is probably also responsible for the reduction of plasma rifampicin concentrations found with coincident administration of para-aminosalicylate (PAS)[9]. If both these drugs are needed, they should be administered at separate times of the day.

Drugs which alter the intestinal flora by an antibacterial action can indirectly influence absorption of other drugs. Much used to be made in this respect of the influence of tetracycline on absorption of B vitamins, although it seems unlikely that the influence is strong. Relative deficiency of vitamin K is produced by gut sterilization with neomycin such that the coumarin anticoagulants probably have an exaggerated action. Furthermore, animal work suggests that methotrexate is normally metabolized by gut flora to the extent that neomycin treatment increases methotrexate lethality[64]. It remains to be seen whether this is also true in man.

Competition for absorption between substances of similar chemical composition is possible theoretically but unproven in practice. It could influence only substances which are actively transported across the intestinal wall. These would include amino acids such as methyldopa and tryptophan and antimetabolites such as azathioprine and methotrexate. Of clinical importance might be the sharing of a transport mechanism between lithium and sodium ions. In theory, absorption of lithium ought to be increased in patients on low salt intake. In practice, lithium treatment is potentially hazardous in this situation but the main site of interaction appears to be renal, competition for tubular reabsorption of sodium and lithium being the deciding factor[50].

Gastrointestinal motility

Drugs which affect gut motility may retard the absorption of other drugs, particularly if they delay gastric emptying. Thus anticholinergic drugs such as atropine derivatives, antispasmodics, phenothiazines and tricyclic antidepressants must delay the appearance of other drugs in the small intestine and their subsequent absorption. Although easily demonstrable in animals, no investigation of this phenomenon appears to have been carried out in man. By contrast, it seems likely that gross intestinal hurry may decrease the absorption of drugs, at least partly because of failure of tablet dissolution in the lumen. This would be of particular importance with enteric-coated preparations and slow-release tablets, absorption from which tends to be rather poor[15].

Intestinal absorptive function

Little is known of individual variability in gastrointestinal absorption beyond those factors already discussed. Frank malabsorption syndromes affect drugs in the same way as essential foodstuffs, vitamins and trace elements. Thus it has been reported that on similar dosage schedules steady-state plasma concentrations of digoxin are lower than in patients with normal absorptive function[30]. This suggests that in malabsorption syndromes the normal degree of digoxin absorption — 80 per cent according to Doherty, Perkins and Mitchell[19], but probably less with many available preparations — is grossly reduced. In two of the patients reported the daily dose of digoxin had to be doubled before steady-state values fell within the normal therapeutic range.

It is apparent from many of the studies reported that there is much individual variability in drug absorption even when all known interfering factors are excluded. In their study of paracetamol absorption, Gwilt and his colleagues[28] found significant differences in absorption from identical preparations under identical conditions. Furthermore, the variation between individuals was such as to suggest that different patients may not necessarily respond in similar fashion to the administration of different commercial products. Variability is also seen in the absorption of phenacetin[32] and propranolol[27], in both cases with considerable resultant differences in plasma drug concentrations. In the case of propranolol, some of the variability may be the result of variations in first-pass metabolism (see Chapter 5), but this is unlikely to account for the differences found with phenacetin. Further investigation is obviously needed.

References

1. Avakian, S. and Kabacoff, B. L. (1964). 'Enhancement of blood antibiotic levels through the combined oral administration of phenethicillin and chymotrypsin.' *Clin. Pharmac. Ther.* **5**, 716—720

2. Barr, W. H., Adir, J. and Garrettson, L. (1971). 'Decrease of tetracycline absorption in man by sodium bicarbonate.' *Clin. Pharmac. Ther.* **12**, 779—784

3. Barr, W. H., Gerbracht, L. M., Letcher, K., Plaut, M. and Strahl, N. (1972). 'Assessment of the biologic availability of tetracycline products in man.' *Clin. Pharmac. Ther.* **13**, 97—108

4. Bauer, G., Rieckmann, P. and Schaumann, W. (1962). 'Einfluss von Teilchengrösse und Lösungsvermittlern auf die Resorption von Spironolacton aus dem Magen-Darmtrakt.' *Arzneimittel-Forsch.* **12**, 487—489

5. Bergman, A. B. and Werner, R. J. (1963). 'Failure of children to receive penicillin by mouth.' *New Engl. J. Med.* **268**, 1334—1338

6. Berry, D., Ross, A. and Deuschle, K. (1963). 'Tuberculous patients treated at home. Comparison of regular and irregular self-medication groups.' *Am. Rev. resp. Dis.* **88**, 769—772

7. Binns, T. B. (Ed.) (1964). *Absorption and Distribution of Drugs.* Edinburgh and London: Churchill Livingstone

8. Blair, D. C. Barnes, R. W., Wildner, E. L. and Murray, W. J. (1971). 'Biological availability of oxytetracycline HCl capsules. A

comparison of all manufacturing sources supplying the United States market.' *J. Am. med. Ass.* **215**, 251–254

9. Boman, G., Hanngren, Å., Malmborg, A-S., Borgå, O. and Sjöqvist, F. (1971). 'Drug interaction: decreased serum concentrations of rifampicin when given with P.A.S.' *Lancet* **1**, 800

10. Bonnar, J., Goldberg, A. and Smith, J. A. (1969). 'Do pregnant women take their iron?' *Lancet* **1**, 457–458

11. Brice, G. W. and Hammer, H. F. (1969). 'Therapeutic nonequivalence of oxytetracycline capsules.' *J. Am. med. Ass.* **208**, 1189–1190

12. Brodie, B. B. (1964). 'Physico-chemical factors in drug absorption.' In *Absorption and Distribution of Drugs*, p. 16. Ed. by T. B. Binns. Edinburgh and London: Churchill Livingstone

13. Campagna, F. A., Cureton, G., Mirigian, R. A. and Nelson, E. (1963). 'Inactive prednisone tablets USP XVI.' *J. pharm. Sci.* **52**, 605–606

14. Cromie, B. W. (1963). 'The feet of clay of the double-blind trial.' *Lancet* **2**, 994–997

15. Crosland-Taylor, P., Keeling, D. H. and Cromie, B. W. (1965). 'A trial of slow-release tablets of ferrous sulphate.' *Curr. ther. Res.* **7**, 244–248

16. Crounse, R. G. (1961). 'Human pharmacology of griseofulvin: the effect of fat intake on gastrointestinal absorption.' *J. invest. Derm.* **37**, 529–532

17. Decker, W. J., Shpall, R. A., Corby, D. G., Combs, H. F. and Payne, C. E. (1969). 'Inhibition of aspirin absorption by activated charcoal and apomorphine.' *Clin. Pharmac. Ther.* **10**, 710–713

18. Dixon, W. M., Stradling, P. and Wooton, I. D. P. (1957). 'Outpatient P.A.S. therapy.' *Lancet* **2**, 871–872

19. Doherty, J. E., Perkins, W. H. and Mitchell, G. K. (1961). 'Tritiated digoxin studies in human subjects.' *Archs intern. Med.* **108**, 531–539

20. Downer, H. D., Galloway, R. W., Horwich, L. and Parke, D. V. (1970). 'The absorption and excretion of carbenoxolone in man.' *J. Pharm. Pharmac.* **22**, 479–487

21. Fraser, E. J., Leach, R. H. and Poston, J. W. (1972). 'Bioavailability of digoxin.' *Lancet* **2**, 541

22. Freestone, D. S. (1969). 'Formulation and therapeutic efficacy of drugs used in clinical trials.' *Lancet* **2**, 98–99

23. Gallo, D. G., Bailey, K. R. and Sheffner, A. L. (1965). 'The interaction between cholestyramine and drugs.' *Proc. Soc. exp. Biol. Med.* **120**, 60–65

24. Glazko, A. J., Kinkel, A. W., Alegnani, W. C. and Holmes, E. L. (1968). 'An evaluation of the absorption characteristics of different chloramphenicol preparations in normal human subjects.' *Clin. Pharmac. Ther.* **9**, 472–483

25. Goldstein, A., Aronow, L. and Kalman, S. M. (1968). *Principles of Drug Action.* New York: Hoeber; London: Harper & Row

26. Goodier, T. E. W., Horwich, L. and Galloway, R. W. (1967). 'Morphological observations on gastric ulcers treated with carbenoxolone sodium.' *Gut* **8**, 544–547

27. Grant, R. H. E., Keelan, P., Kernohan, R. J., Leonard, J. C., Nancekievill, L. and Sinclair, K. (1966). 'Multicenter trial of propranolol in angina pectoris.' *Am. J. Cardiol.* **18**, 361–365

28. Gwilt, J. R., Robertson, A., Goldman, L. and Blanchard, A. W. (1963). 'The absorption characteristics of paracetamol tablets in man.' *J. Pharm. Pharmac.* **15**, 445–453

29. Hahn, K.-J., Eiden, W., Schettle, M., Hahn, M., Walter, E. and Weber, E. (1972). 'Effect of cholestyramine on the gastrointestinal absorption of phenprocoumon and acetylsalicylic acid in man.' *Eur. J. clin. Pharmac.* **4**, 142–145

30. Heizer, W. D., Smith, T. W. and Goldfinger, S. E. (1971). 'Absorption of digoxin in patients with malabsorption syndromes.' *New Engl. J. Med.* **285**, 257–259

31. Joyce, C. R. B. (1962). 'Patient co-operation and the sensitivity of clinical trials.' *J. chron. Dis.* **15**, 1025–1036

32. Kampffmeyer, H. G. (1971). 'Elimination of phenacetin and phenazone by man before and after treatment with phenobarbital.' *Eur. J. clin. Pharmac.* **3**, 113–118

33. Kerr, D. N. S. and Davidson, S. (1958). 'The prophylaxis of iron-deficiency anaemia in pregnancy.' *Lancet* **2**, 483–488

34. Knudsen, E. T., Brown, D. M. and Rolinson, G. N. (1962). 'A new orally effective penicillinase-stable penicillin – BRL.1621.' *Lancet* **2**, 632–634

35. Kunin, C. M. and Finland, M. (1961). 'Clinical pharmacology of the tetracycline antibiotics.' *Clin. Pharmac. Ther.* **2**, 51–69

36. Leading Article (1968). 'Iron in flour.' *Lancet* **2**, 495–497

37. Leonards, J. R. (1963). 'The influence of solubility on the rate of gastrointestinal absorption of aspirin.' *Clin. Pharmac. Ther.* **4**, 476–479

38. Levy, G., Leonards, J. R. and Procknal, J. A. (1965). 'Development of *in vitro* dissolution tests which correlate quantitatively with dissolution rate-limited drug absorption in man.' *J. pharm. Sci.* **54**, 1719–1722

39. Levy, G. and Tsuchiya, T. (1972). 'Effect of activated charcoal on aspirin absorption in man.' *Clin. Pharmac. Ther.* **13**, 317–322

40. Lindenbaum, J., Mellow, M. H., Blackstone, M. O. and Butler, V. P. (1971). 'Variation in biologic availability of digoxin from four preparations.' *New Engl. J. Med.* **285**, 1344–1347

41. Luntz, G. R. W. N. and Asutin, R. (1960). 'New stick test for P.A.S. in urine. Report on use of "Phenistix" and problems of long-term chemotherapy for tuberculosis.' *Br. med. J.* **1**, 1679–1684

42. McCarthy, C. G. and Finland, M. (1960). 'Absorption and excretion of four penicillins, penicillin G, penicillin V, phenethicillin and phenylmercaptomethylpenicillin.' *New Engl. J. Med.* **263**, 315–326

43. McGilveray, I. J. and Mattock, G. L. (1972). 'Some factors affecting the absorption of paracetamol.' *J. Pharm. Pharmac.* **24**, 615–619

44. McMartin, C. and Simpson, P. (1971). 'The absorption and metabolism of guanethidine in hypertensive patients requiring different doses of the drug.' *Clin. Pharmac. Ther.* **12**, 73–77

45. Manninen, V., Melin, J. and Härtel, G. (1971). 'Serum-digoxin concentrations during treatment with different preparations.' *Lancet* **2**, 934–935

46. Manninen, V., Melin, J. and Reissel, P. (1972). 'Tablet disintegration: possible link with biological availability of digoxin.' *Lancet* **1**, 490–491

47. Mohler, D. N., Wallin, D. G. and Dreyfus, E. G. (1955). 'Studies in the home treatment of streptococcal disease. I. Failure of patients to take penicillin by mouth as prescribed.' *New Engl. J. Med.* **252**, 1116–1118

48. O'Reilly, R. A. and Aggeler, P. M. (1969). 'Effect of barbiturates on oral anticoagulants in man.' *Clin. Res.* **17**, 153

49. Pickering, G. W., Cranston, W. I. and Pears, M. A. (1961). *The Treatment of Hypertension.* Springfield, Ill: Thomas

50. Platman, S. F. and Fieve, R. R. (1969). 'Lithium retention and excretion.' *Archs gen. Psychiat.* **20**, 285–289

51. Porter, A. M. W. (1969). 'Drug defaulting in a general practice.' *Br. med. J.* **1**, 218–222

52. Robinson, D. S., Benjamin, D. M. and McCormack, J. J. (1971). 'Interaction of warfarin and nonsystemic gastrointestinal drugs.' *Clin. Pharmac. Ther.* **12**, 491–495

53. Searl, R. O. and Pernarowski, M. (1967). 'The biopharmaceutical properties of solid dosage forms: I. An evaluation of 23 brands of phenylbutazone tablets.' *Can. med. Ass. J.* **96**, 1513–1520

54. Shaw, T. R. D., Howard, M. R. and Hamer, J. (1972). 'Variation in the biological availability of digoxin.' *Lancet* **2**, 303–307

55. Stewart, R. B. and Cluff, L. E. (1972). 'A review of medication errors and compliance in ambulant patients.' *Clin. Pharmac. Ther.* **13**, 463–468

56. Sutherland, R., Croydon, E. A. P. and Rolinson, G. N. (1970). 'Flucloxacillin, a new isoxazolyl penicillin, compared with oxacillin, cloxacillin, and dicloxacillin.' *Br. med. J.* **4**, 455–460

57. Tannenbaum, P. J., Rosen, E., Flanagan, T. and Crosley, A. P. (1968). 'The influence of dosage form on the activity of a diuretic agent.' *Clin. Pharmac. Ther.* **9**, 598–604

58. Tyrer, J. H., Eadie, M. J., Sutherland, J. M. and Hooper, W. D. (1970). 'Outbreak of anticonvulsant intoxication in an Australian city.' *Br. med. J.* **4**, 271–273

59. Varley, A. B. (1968). 'The generic inequivalence of drugs.' *J. Am. med. Ass.* **206**, 1745–1748

60. Vere, D. W. (1965). 'Errors of complex prescribing.' *Lancet* **1**, 370–373

61. Wagner, J. G. (1961). 'Biopharmaceutics: absorption aspects.' *J. pharm. Sci.* **50**, 359–387

62. Wagner, J. G., Gerard, E. S. and Kaiser, D. G. (1966).. 'The effect of the dosage form on serum levels of indoxole.' *Clin. Pharmac. Ther.* **7**, 610–619

63. Wagner, J. G., Welling, P. G., Lee, K. P. and Walker, J. E. (1971). '*In vivo* and *in vitro* availability of commercial warfarin tablets.' *J. pharm. Sci.* **60**, 666–677

64. Zaharko, D. A., Bruckner, H. and Oliverio, V. T. (1969). 'Antibiotics alter methotrexate metabolism and excretion.' *Science, N.Y.* **166**, 887–888

CHAPTER 4

Drug Distribution

Once a drug has entered the circulation, it may gain access to a variety of 'compartments' within the body. For most drugs this distribution occurs by diffusion from regions of high to regions of low concentration. Volatile anaesthetics are, however, distributed according to partial pressure gradients rather than concentration gradients. The rate and extent of drug distribution depends principally on:

(1) the physicochemical properties of the drug, particularly its lipid solubility;

(2) the regional distribution of blood flow to the various tissues and organs of the body;

(3) the binding of drugs to proteins and other body constituents;

(4) the active transport of a few drugs across cell membranes.

The plasma concentration of a drug, whether given as a single dose or after multiple dosing, depends in part on its apparent volume of distribution (see Chapter 2). Variability of this volume therefore contributes to variability of plasma concentrations both between and within individuals. A few drugs are distributed within a strict anatomical space such as plasma water (0.05 l/kg), extracellular water (0.17 l/kg) or total body water (0.60 l/kg). Drugs distributed in this manner such as heparin (in plasma), thiocyanate (in extracellular water) and antipyrine (in total body water) show little interindividual variation in apparent volume of distribution. Such variability as is observed is due to the fact that in obese people a larger fraction of body weight is fat, so that the fluid compartments all represent smaller proportions of the body weight. In infants, the total body water (0.80 l/kg) represents a larger proportion of the body weight, at least partly because the bony tissues are incompletely calcified and therefore contribute less to body weight than in adults.

For drugs which are not uniformly distributed, marked interindividual differences may be demonstrated. The origin of this variability is unclear. The observation that identical twins have similar but fraternal twins dissimilar apparent distribution volumes of nortriptyline[2] indicates that it may be partly genetic in origin. Diazepam distribution volumes have been found to vary sevenfold between individuals[72] and such variations must have a profound influence on plasma concentrations of this drug, but why such differences should pertain to diazepam, and not to many other drugs (Table 4.1), is completely unknown at present.

TABLE 4.1. Range of Apparent Distribution Volumes of Some Drugs in Normal Subjects

Drug	Range of apparent distribution volume (l/kg)	Reference
Antipyrine	0.48−0.70	−
Amylobarbitone	0.5−1.1 (approx.)	[47]
Diazepam	0.18−1.30	[72]
Growth hormone	0.071−0.093	[70]
Heparin	0.055−0.059	[24]
Insulin	0.054−0.112	[70]
Lignocaine	0.58−1.91	[60]
Nalidixic acid	0.26−0.45	[55]
Nortriptyline	22.5−56.9	[2]
Phenylbutazone	0.04−0.15	−
Procainamide	1.74−2.22	[36]
Theophylline	0.33−0.74	[35]
Warfarin	0.09−0.24	−

The concurrent administration of other drugs and the presence of disease are potential sources of further variability in apparent distribution volume but have again been the subject of little investigation. Gibaldi and Schwartz[28] have shown that the administration of probenecid not only inhibits the renal excretion but also reduces the apparent distribution volumes of ampicillin and cephaloridine. The mechanism by which this occurs is unknown but could be due to competition either for tissue-binding sites or for transport mechanisms. Altered drug distribution volumes have also been found in various disease states; e.g. procainamide in cardiac failure[36], amylobarbitone[47] and growth hormone[70] in liver disease, and insulin in diabetes[70]. Such variability may well account in part for the variability in drug response which is found in these conditions. Changes in drug distribution have also been suggested to account for the variation in digoxin sensitivity in patients with thyroid disease[19]; hyperthyroid patients were found to have consistently lower, and hypothyroid patients higher, plasma digoxin concentrations than had euthyroid patients after similar drug doses. Drug elimination rates were similar in the three groups.

Lipid solubility

In order for a drug to leave the circulation it must penetrate the capillary endothelial lining. With the exception of those in the brain, capillary membranes are generally freely permeable to most drugs which therefore gain ready access to the extracellular space. In the brain, however, the tight 'junctions' between capillary endothelial cells constitute an important barrier to the diffusion of compounds into the central nervous system. Compounds entering both the brain (from the circulation) and the tissue cells (from the extracellular space) must cross lipoprotein cell membranes which are most easily penetrated by lipid-soluble drugs. Most drugs, being weak electrolytes, exist in both ionized and non-ionized forms, only the latter having significant lipid solubility. The ease and extent to which a drug can cross cell membranes is therefore dependent on its pK_a value (ionization constant) and on the pH of its solution. Weakly acidic drugs such as salicylates are less ionized, and therefore more lipid-soluble, at low pH; hence the ease with which they penetrate into the cells of the gastric mucosa. Weakly basic drugs such as amphetamines are more ionized, and therefore less lipid-soluble, at low pH.

The pK_a values of a large number of commonly used drugs are shown in Appendix C. From such data it would be predicted that those drugs which are least ionized at physiological pH would diffuse most rapidly into the central nervous system. This prediction has been confirmed experimentally[11].

Sudden changes in acid–base balance alter extracellular pH more readily than intracellular pH. A fall in plasma pH leads to an increase in the non-ionized fraction of acidic drugs and a decrease in the non-ionized fraction of basic drugs. This results in a fall in the plasma concentration and a rise in the tissue level of an acidic drug and the converse in the case of basic drugs. It has been shown that in dogs[73] respiratory acidosis produced by CO_2 ventilation results in a fall in plasma phenobarbitone (an acidic drug) and an increase in both tissue phenobarbitone level and the depth of anaesthesia. Thus the therapeutic value of treating patients suffering from phenobarbitone poisoning with intravenous bicarbonate (to alkalinize the urine) may depend, in part at least, on reversing this gradient.

Regional blood flow

The uptake of a drug by an organ is partly determined by its blood flow and its tissue mass. On the basis of perfusion characteristics, the tissues of the body can be divided into four groups[59]:

(1)   well perfused, lean tissues including the heart, lungs, kidneys, brain, endocrine and exocrine glands;
(2)   moderately perfused, lean tissues including muscle and skin;
(3)   fat;
(4)   negligibly perfused tissues including bone, teeth, tendons and ligaments.

Other factors being equal, well perfused tissues in group 1 will equilibrate rapidly with plasma by comparison with tissues in group 2. Voluntary muscle in the latter group equilibrates at only a moderate rate, although its capacity for drug uptake is quite large because of its mass. The adipose tissue of group 3 is rather poorly perfused but it represents an important depot for lipid-soluble drugs which is subject to considerable interindividual variation. Thus in lean persons it represents only 10 per cent of body weight; in obesity the proportion is much greater, perhaps even 50 per cent *in extremis*. The interplay between the various tissue groups is reflected in the fate of intravenous thiopentone, which is sequentially distributed to tissues according to their perfusion characteristics[31, 56]. Its final disposition must inevitably be affected by the size of the fat depot mass.

Fat itself does not appear to be entirely homogeneous with respect to drug distribution[54]. Some agents, anaesthetic gases in particular, are apparently capable of diffusing into adipose tissue directly from adjacent, highly perfused lean tissues. Perirenal fat and omental fat are able to accumulate some anaesthetic gases to a greater degree than is subcutaneous fat.

Whether disturbances of regional blood flow are responsible for important changes in drug distribution in clinical medicine is unproven though probable. The increased volume of distribution of penicillin in recumbency[40] may be explicable on this basis, and the changes in distribution of procainamide and lignocaine in heart failure, digoxin in thyroid disease, amylobarbitone in liver disease and insulin in diabetes (see above) might also be due to changes in regional blood flow.

Binding of drugs

Many drugs bind reversibly to tissues or plasma proteins and the importance of this process lies in the fact that only the unbound fraction is freely available for distribution, elimination or combination with receptor sites.

Plasma protein binding of drugs

In plasma, the most important contribution to drug binding is made by albumin. This process is reversible and can be represented thus[30] :

$$\text{drug} + \text{protein} \mathrel{\mathop{\rightleftharpoons}^{k_1}_{k_2}} \text{drug–protein complex}$$

The extent to which a drug is bound is dependent on the following.

(1) The association constant (K_A). – The ratio of the rate constants of association (k_1) and dissociation (k_2) is the association constant (K_A). This is a measure of the affinity of drug for protein; the higher the association constant the tighter the binding.

(2) The number of binding sites. – Whilst the precise nature of the binding forces between drugs and plasma proteins is uncertain, only a few (and often one or two) drug molecules can bind to each molecule. The number of binding sites, however, varies for different drugs.

(3) The protein concentration. – Changes in the concentration of albumin alter the number of binding sites available for drug combination. The fraction of drug which is bound, therefore, increases with albumin concentration *(Figure 4.1)*.

(4) The drug concentration. – Increasing drug concentration results in a fall in the fraction of drug bound due to partial saturation of the binding sites. Although a graph relating these variables is non-linear *(Figure 4.2)*, at therapeutic drug concentrations the proportion of drug bound is roughly constant because the concentrations fall on the left-hand, linear, part of the curve.

Although in plasma a drug may be highly bound to protein the total amount so bound is not necessarily a large proportion of all the drug in the body. Reference to Table 4.1 shows that nortriptyline, for example,

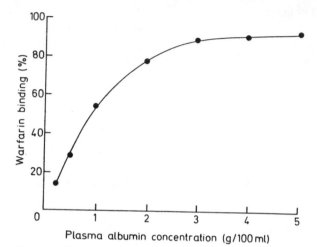

Figure 4.1. Effect of increasing albumin concentration on the degree of binding of warfarin. (From O'Reilly, 1967[53])

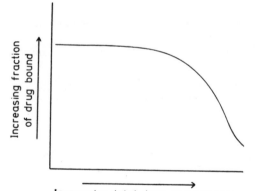

Figure 4.2. Effect of increasing drug concentration on the binding of drug to plasma proteins

has a huge distribution volume and consequently less than 1 per cent of all the drug in the body at steady-state is present in the plasma. The fact that this drug is highly bound to plasma protein, therefore, is unlikely to be of much consequence. By contrast, the large degree of protein binding shown by warfarin must be of considerable importance because as much as 50 per cent of this drug may be present in the plasma due to its small distribution volume.

Plasma protein binding has important consequences for drug absorption, distribution and elimination. Drug absorption is assisted because diffusion across the intestinal wall continues as long as the concentration within the gut exceeds that of the unbound fraction within the

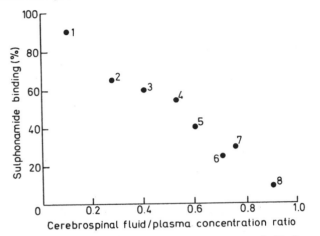

Figure 4.3. Relationship between percentage protein binding and the c.s.f. plasma concentration ratios of various sulphonamides:

(1) sulphamethoxypyridazine   (5) sulphadiazine
(2) sulphamethoxazole   (6) sulphathiazole
(3) sulphadimidine   (7) sulphapyridine
(4) sulphamethoxydiazine   (8) sulphanilamide
    (Based on data from Garrod and O'Grady, 1971[27])

capillaries. Similarly, only unbound drug in the plasma is available for distribution; other factors being equal the greater the degree of binding the less will be the tissue concentration relative to the total (bound plus unbound) plasma concentration. The relationship between the degree of binding of various sulphonamides and the cerebrospinal fluid (c.s.f.) to total plasma concentration ratios attained is shown in *Figure 4.3*. It can be seen that sulphonamides which are highly bound to albumin are less able to gain access to c.s.f. than those whose binding is less. Further illustration is provided by the fact that in epileptic patients c.s.f. concentrations of phenytoin show close agreement with the unbound, but not with the total plasma concentrations[46]. The importance of protein binding on drug distribution is also demonstrated by the use of diazoxide. Given intravenously, this compound is a valuable hypotensive agent in the treatment of accelerated hypertension. It is extensively bound to plasma albumin and if administered by a slow infusion (over 100 seconds) the hypotensive response is disappointing[50, 61] because most of the drug becomes protein-bound and is unable to reach the arteriolar walls. Rapid intravenous administration (less than 10 seconds) produces a 'bolus' of diazoxide in which (for probably no more than one or two circulation times) the unbound fraction of drug is high; the drug is available at this time to diffuse into the arteriolar walls and cause a fall in peripheral vascular tone.

Since only the unbound fraction of any drug in the plasma is available for metabolism or excretion, appreciable binding results in delayed elimination. This is illustrated by the differing rates of elimination of digitoxin and digoxin; both are bound exclusively to albumin, but at therapeutic plasma levels the unbound fraction is 5 per cent for digitoxin and 77 per cent for digoxin. As a result, digitoxin is less available for metabolism and therefore has a longer half-life[45].

Plasma protein-binding characteristics of a number of commonly used drugs are indicated in Appendix C.

The foregoing account would suggest that reductions in the binding of drugs to plasma proteins might result in a variety of unwanted effects. In hypoproteinaemic disorders (such as the nephrotic syndrome, liver disease, coeliac disease and starvation), a rise in the unbound fraction could lead to changes in the efficacy and toxicity of a given drug dose. At the same time drug elimination would inevitably increase so that efficacy and toxicity might be reduced. Clearly, however, such influences are likely to be important only for drugs which are extensively bound to plasma proteins and which have a small volume of distribution. Patients with the nephrotic syndrome eliminate the dye Evans blue more rapidly than normals[76], and relative resistance to warfarin has been described in a nephrotic patient (plasma albumin: 1.6 g/100 ml) in whom warfarin elimination was 10.7 per cent/hour as opposed to the normal 1.6 per cent/hour[42]. Hypoalbuminaemia (less than 2.5 g/100 ml) is associated with a twofold increase in the frequency of side-effects from prednisone therapy[41] which is possibly due to the fact that prednisolone, the active metabolite of prednisone, is normally largely bound to albumin. Finally, the reduced protein binding of drugs in neonates is, in part, due to the low plasma albumin at this stage of development[22].

Whilst it is clear that quantitative changes in plasma proteins lead to changes in drug binding, it has recently become apparent that qualitative differences may also be important. Curry[17] has shown that the unbound fraction of chlorpromazine varies from 1 to 10 per cent between individuals, although there are no significant interindividual differences in the protein binding of desipramine[7] or phenytoin[68]. There are interindividual differences in protein binding of nortriptyline which appear, from a recent twin study, to be partially under genetic control[3].

Plasma from patients with renal failure shows diminished binding of sulphonamides[5], digitoxin[64] and phenytoin[58]. This is due partly to the hypoalbuminaemia which may occur in such patients but also to qualitative changes in the binding proteins themselves. The diminished binding of phenytoin may explain why uraemic patients have low steady-state plasma concentrations[38] and why they respond to treatment at such low levels[52]. Protein binding of desipramine is unaltered in this disorder[58], indicating that the influence is not ubiquitous.

Many drugs share binding sites on plasma proteins with other drugs or with endogenous substances such as uric acid, bilirubin and certain hormones. The displacement of hormones from their carrier proteins does not appear to be of importance. Thus, phenytoin, although lowering protein-bound iodine[75], does not produce clinical hypothyroidism or significant change in radioiodine uptake by the thyroid gland, and cessation of therapy is followed by a return of the protein-bound iodine value to normal[71]. A number of anti-inflammatory drugs including salicylates, phenylbutazone and indomethacin displace cortisol from globulin[9] without apparent ill-effect. By contrast, the interaction between acidic drugs and bilirubin is of considerable importance, at least during the neonatal period. First, the presence of bilirubin reduces drug binding, either by reducing the number of available binding sites[22] or by reducing the affinity of the protein for the drug[13]. Secondly, some drugs displace bilirubin from binding sites; this results in an increase in the unbound bilirubin fraction in the plasma which is then available to cross the poorly developed blood—brain barrier of infants and produce kernicterus. This interaction emerged during a clinical trial of the comparative efficacy of tetracycline and a sulphonamide mixture in the management of premature infants[65]. The sulphonamide mixture led to a significantly higher mortality, and kernicterus was found at autopsy.

Competition between different drugs for the same binding sites on plasma has been thought to be of considerable practical importance because the unbound fraction of the drug displaced from its protein would increase and thereby have an enhanced pharmacological effect. Thus sulphinpyrazone (a potent uricosuric agent) displaces sulphamethoxypyridazine from albumin in rats, with a fall in the total plasma concentration and an increase in the tissue level of the latter drug[4]

(Figure 4.4). In man, Kunin[37] has shown that sulphamethoxy-pyridazine, sulphaethylthiadazole and acetylsalicylic acid reduce penicillin binding to plasma proteins *in vitro,* and *in vivo* cause a fall in total serum penicillin and a rise in the free (unbound) fraction.

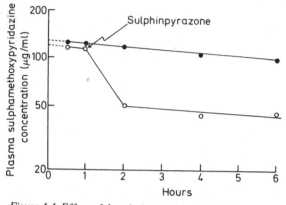

Figure 4.4. *Effect of the administration of sulphinpyrazone on the plasma decline of sulphamethoxypyridazine in rats. (From Anton, 1961[4])*

Because of the potential importance of displacement, many *in vitro* studies have been undertaken in order to predict possible interactions between protein-bound drugs *in vivo.* Such investigations have predictive value only if the drug to be displaced has a small distribution volume (see above). In such a circumstance, if the drug is extensively protein-bound and has a low therapeutic ratio (e.g. coumarin anticoagulants and oral hypoglycaemic agents), its displacement from a binding site might be of considerable consequence. By contrast, displacement of a drug with a large distribution volume would be unimportant because the displaced drug molecules would be distributed so widely that the concentration of drug at its site of action (or elimination) would be virtually unaltered.

In vitro studies have shown that clofibrate[68], phenylbutazone[69], nalidixic acid, ethacrynic acid and diazoxide[62] can displace warfarin from binding sites. Similarly, salicylates, sulphonamides and phenylbutazone[14, 69] displace sulphonylurea hypoglycaemic drugs. *In vivo,* increased anticoagulation has been observed in patients on warfarin after the administration of phenylbutazone[23], oxyphenbutazone[33] and clofibrate[32]. The interaction between phenylbutazone and warfarin appears to be due to displacement from binding sites[1] but the mechanism by which clofibrate interacts with warfarin is less clear since this drug may also increase the affinity of the receptor for warfarin in the liver[68]. The mechanism by which certain sulphonamides potentiate the hypoglycaemic effect of tolbutamide is also confused. Whilst both sulphaphenazole and sulphadimethoxine can displace tolbutamide from plasma protein *in vitro,* only the former precipitates hypoglycaemia *in vivo*[14]. Sellers and Koch-Weser[63] found that chloral hydrate potentiated the anticoagulant action of warfarin in 25 per cent of hospitalized patients receiving this combination. The explanation appears to be that bound warfarin is displaced from protein-binding sites by trichloroacetic acid, the major metabolite of chloral hydrate[62]. At the present time, therefore, the only drug interactions proven to be due to displacement from plasma-protein-binding sites are those of warfarin and phenylbutazone and warfarin and trichloroacetic acid.

It is of interest to note that some drugs apparently increase the protein binding of other drugs. Thus pempidine, which is not normally protein bound, becomes extensively bound *in vitro* in the presence of chlorothiazide[8, 21]. Similarly, tetracyclines increase the binding of both promazine and chlorpromazine to albumin[26]. The practical implication of these findings is not yet clear.

Tissue binding of drugs

The relatively large distribution volumes of drugs such as nortriptyline (see Table 4.1) can only be accounted for by extensive binding in tissues. Similarly, the high tissue/plasma concentration ratios for digoxin (30:1)[20] and quinine (20:1)[16] also emphasize the considerable degree of tissue binding that may occur. Despite this, the ability of tissues to bind drugs is largely unexplored although tissue homogenates have been shown to bind barbiturates[29], phenothiazines, procainamide and phenylbutazone by different mechanisms[9]. One possible interaction between drugs bound to tissue proteins has been described for pamaquin and mepacrine[77]. When the former drug is given to patients previously treated with mepacrine, the pamaquin is inadequately bound to tissues and its plasma concentration is five- to tenfold greater with an associated increase in toxicity.

Tissue binding of drugs is being increasingly recognized as an important mechanism for the production of adverse reactions to drugs and chemicals. Tetracyclines chelate with newly laid down bone, producing a tetracycline-calcium orthophosphate complex. The half-life of tetracycline in bone is of the order of several months[12]. In adults, this appears to be of little importance but in neonates a 40 per cent depression of bone growth has been demonstrated following tetracycline administration[15]. They are deposited also in foetal teeth following administration to the mother during pregnancy, with subsequent enamel hypoplasia, cusp malformation, yellow or brown pigmentation and increased susceptibility to caries.

A number of polycyclic aromatic compounds such as chloroquine and phenothiazines interact with melanin. *In vivo,* high concentrations of these drugs accumulate in the melanin-containing tissues of the eye, suggesting a relationship to the retinopathies produced by these drugs[6]. Recent studies have also indicated that the hepatotoxicity of certain compounds such as carbon tetrachloride, bromobenzene[10] and phenacetin[49] derives from the fact that they are oxidized in the liver (see Chapter 5) to active 'intermediates' (probably epoxides) which bind covalently to macromolecules in the liver and cause hepatic necrosis.

Active transport of drugs

Whilst the distribution of most drugs occurs by passive diffusion, a few drugs which resemble physiological compounds undergo active transport through certain cellular membranes. Thus the adrenergic neurone-blocking agents guanethidine, bethanidine and debrisoquine are believed to gain access to sympathetic nerve terminals by means of the amine transport system[34]. Tricyclic antidepressants, phenothiazines and cocaine, which are potent antagonists of amine transport, antagonize also the hypotensive actions of the adrenergic neurone-blocking agents[25, 39, 48, 67]. This particular drug interaction, therefore, presumably arises because the antihypertensive agent no longer gains access to the nerve terminals. Since depression is not uncommon in patients receiving hypotensive therapy this interaction is particularly unfortunate. If antidepressant therapy is necessary, thiazide diuretics in combination with a beta-adrenoceptor-blocking agent[66] are the drugs of choice in managing the hypertension.

There is increasing evidence that certain organic anions are actively transported from c.s.f. into plasma at the choroid plexus[18]. This pump removes 5-hydroxyindolylacetic acid[51] and salicylate[44] from the c.s.f. and is inhibited by organic acids such as perchlorate and probenecid. It is possible that significant increases in the c.s.f. concentration of penicillins (also acidic drugs) could be achieved by concurrent administration of probenecid to patients with meningitis[57]. It has also recently been shown that, in rabbits at least, morphine is actively transported into the c.s.f. from plasma and that this process can be inhibited by structurally related bases such as codeine and nalorphine[74].

Placental drug transfer

Placental transfer of drugs from mother to foetus occurs predominantly by simple diffusion. Lipid solubility, pK_a and protein binding (in both mother and foetus) play important roles in determining the rate and extent of this process. In addition, it is known that active transport of certain endogenous compounds, including vitamins, amino acids, inorganic ions and pyrimidines, occurs. Drugs having structural similarities to these endogenous materials may cross the placenta by such mechanisms, producing high foetal:maternal concentration ratios. Studies indicate that 5-fluorouracil (a pyrimidine analogue)[43] and methyldopa (an amino acid) may be so affected.

References

1. Aggeler, P. M., O'Reilly, R. A., Leong, L. and Kowitz, P. E. (1967). 'Potentiation of anticoagulant effect of warfarin by phenylbutazone.' *New Engl. J. Med.* **276**, 496–501
2. Alexanderson, B. (1972). 'On interindividual variability in plasma levels of nortriptyline and desmethylimipramine in man: a pharmacokinetic and genetic study.' *Linköping Univ. Med. Dissertations* No. 6, Linköping, Sweden
3. Alexanderson, B. and Borgå, O. (1972). 'Interindividual differences in plasma protein binding of nortriptyline in man – a twin study.' *Eur. J. clin. Pharmac.* **4**, 196–200
4. Anton, A. H. (1961). 'A drug-induced change in the distribution and renal excretion of sulfonamides.' *J. Pharmac. exp. Ther.* **134**, 291–303
5. Anton, A. H. and Corey, W. J. (1971). 'Plasma protein binding of sulfonamides in anephric patients.' *Fedn Proc.* **30**, 629
6. Bernstein, H., Zvaifler, N., Rubin, M. and Mansour, A. M. (1963). 'The ocular deposition of chloroquine.' *Invest. Ophthalmol.* **2**, 384–392
7. Borgå, O., Azarnoff, D. Z., Plym Forshell, G. and Sjöqvist, F. (1969). 'Plasma protein binding of tricyclic antidepressants in man.' *Biochem. Pharmac.* **18**, 2135–2143
8. Breckenridge, A. and Rosen, A. (1971). 'The binding of chlorothiazide to plasma proteins.' *Biochim. biophys. Acta* **229**, 610–617
9. Brodie, B. B. (1965). 'Displacement of one drug by another from carrier or receptor sites.' *Proc. R. Soc. Med.* **58**, 946–955
10. Brodie, B. B., Cho, A. K., Krishna, G. and Reid, W. D. (1971). 'Drug metabolism in man: past, present and future.' *Ann. N.Y. Acad. Sci.* **179**, 11–18

11. Brodie, B. B., Kurz, H. and Schanker, L. S. (1960). 'The importance of dissociation constant and lipid solubility in influencing the passage of drugs into the cerebrospinal fluid.' *J. Pharmac. exp. Ther.* **130**, 20—25

12. Buyske, D. A., Eisner, H. J. and Kelly, R. G. (1960). 'Concentration and persistence of tetracycline and chlortetracycline in bone.' *J. Pharmac. exp. Ther.* **130**, 150—156

13. Chignell, C. F., Vesell, E. S., Starkweather, D. K. and Berlin, C. M. (1971). 'The binding of sulfaphenazole to fetal, neonatal, and adult human plasma albumin.' *Clin. Pharmac. Ther.* **12**, 897—901

14. Christensen, L. K., Hansen, J. M. and Kristensen, M. (1963). 'Sulphaphenazole-induced hypoglycaemic attacks in tolbutamide-treated diabetics.' *Lancet* **2**, 1298—1301

15. Cohlan, S. Q., Bevelander, G. and Tiamsic, T. (1963). 'Growth inhibition of prematures receiving tetracyclines: a clinical and laboratory investigation.' *Am. J. Dis. Child.* **105**, 453—461

16. Conn, H. L. and Luchi, R. J. (1964). 'Some cellular and metabolic considerations relating to the action of quinidine as a prototype antiarrhythmic agent.' *Am. J. Med.* **37**, 685—699

17. Curry, S. H. (1970). 'Plasma protein binding of chlorpromazine.' *J. Pharm. Pharmac.* **22**, 193—197

18. Davson, H. (1967). *Physiology of the Cerebrospinal Fluid*. Edinburgh and London: Churchill Livingstone

19. Doherty, J. E. and Perkins, W. H. (1966). 'Digoxin metabolism in hypo- and hyperthyroidism. Studies with tritiated digoxin in thyroid disease.' *Ann. intern. Med.* **64**, 489—507

20. Doherty, J. E., Perkins, W. H. and Flanigan, W. J. (1967). 'The distribution and concentration of tritiated digoxin in human tissues.' *Ann. intern. Med.* **66**, 116—124

21. Dollery, C. T., Emslie-Smith, D. and Muggleton, D. F. (1960). 'Actions of chlorothiazide in hypertension.' *Proc. R. Soc. Med.* **53**, 592—594

22. Ehrnebo, M., Agurell, S., Jalling, B. and Boreus, L. O. (1971). 'Age differences in drug binding by plasma proteins: studies on human foetuses, neonates and adults.' *Eur. J. clin. Pharmac.* **3**, 189—193

23. Eisen, M. J. (1964). 'Combined effect of sodium warfarin and phenylbutazone.' *J. Am. med. Ass.* **189**, 64—65

24. Estes, J. W., Pelikan, E. W. and Krüger-Thiemer, E. (1969). 'A retrospective study of the pharmacokinetics of heparin.' *Clin. Pharmac. Ther.* **10**, 329—339

25. Fann. W. E., Janowsky, D. S., Davis, J. M. and Oates, J. A. (1971). 'Chlorpromazine reversal of the antihypertensive action of guanethidine.' *Lancet* **2**, 436—437

26. Franz, J. W., Jähnchen, E. and Krieglstein, J. (1969). 'Der Einflus verschiedener Pharmaka auf das Bindungsvermögen einer Albu-

minlösung für Promazin und Chlorpromazin.' *Naunyn-Schmiedebergs Arch. exp. Path. Pharmak.* **264**, 462–475

27. Garrod, L. P. and O'Grady, F. (1971). *Antibiotic and Chemotherapy*, 3rd edn. Edinburgh and London: Churchill Livingstone
28. Gibaldi, M. and Schwartz, M. A. (1968). 'Apparent effect of probenecid on the distribution of penicillin in man.' *Clin. Pharmac. Ther.* **9**, 345–349
29. Goldbaum, L. R. and Smith, P. K. (1954). 'The interaction of barbiturates with serum albumin and its possible relation to their disposition and pharmacological action.' *J. Pharmac. exp. Ther.* **111**, 197–209
30. Goldstein, A. (1949). 'The interactions of drugs and plasma proteins.' *Pharmac. Rev.* **1**, 102–165
31. Goldstein, A. and Aronow, L. (1960). 'The duration of action of thiopental and pentobarbital.' *J. Pharmac. exp. Ther.* **128**, 1–6
32. Hellman, L., Zumoff, B., Kessler, G., Kara, E., Rubin, I. L. and Rosenfeld, R. S. (1963). 'Reduction of cholesterol and lipids in man by ethyl-*p*-chlorophenoxy-isobutyrate.' *Ann. intern. Med.* **59**, 477–494
33. Hobbs, C. B., Miller, A. L. and Thornley, J. H. (1965). 'Potentiation of anticoagulant therapy by oxyphenylbutazone.' *Postgrad. med. J.* **41**, 563–565
34. Iversen, L. L. (1967). *The Uptake and Storage of Noradrenaline by Sympathetic Nerves*. Cambridge: University Press
35. Jenne, J. W., Wyze, E., Rood, F. S. and MacDonald, F. M. (1972). 'Pharmacokinetics of theophylline.' *Clin. Pharmac. Ther.* **13**, 349–360
36. Koch-Weser, J. (1971). 'Pharmacokinetics of procainamide in man.' *Ann. N.Y. Acad. Sci.* **179**, 370–382
37. Kunin, C. M. (1966). 'Clinical pharmacology of the new penicillins. II. Effect of drugs which interfere with binding to serum proteins.' *Clin. Pharmac. Ther.* **7**, 180–188
38. Kutt, H. (1971). 'Biochemical and genetic factors regulating Dilantin metabolism in man.' *Ann. N.Y. Acad. Sci.* **179**, 704–722
39. Leishman, A. W. D., Matthews, H. L. and Smith, A. J. (1963). 'Antagonism of guanethidine by imipramine.' *Lancet* **1**, 112
40. Levy, G. (1967). 'Effect of bed rest on distribution and elimination of drugs.' *J. pharm Sci.* **56**, 928–929
41. Lewis, G. P., Jusko, W. J., Burke, C. W. and Graves, L. (1971). 'Prednisone side effects and serum-protein levels.' *Lancet* **2**, 778–781
42. Lewis, R. J., Spivack, M. and Spaet, T. H. (1967). 'Warfarin resistance.' *Am. J. Med.* **42**, 620–624
43. Long, R. F. and Marks, J. (1969). 'The transfer of drugs across the placenta.' *Proc. R. Soc. Med.* **62**, 318–321

44.   Lorenzo, A. V. and Spector, R. (1972). 'The uptake of salicylic acid by choroid plexus.' *Fedn Proc.* **31**, 604

45.   Lukas, D. S. and De Martino, A. G. (1969). 'Binding of digitoxin and some related cardenolides to human plasma proteins.' *J. clin. Invest.* **48**, 1041–1053

46.   Lund, L., Berlin, A. and Lunde, P. K. M. (1972). 'Plasma binding of diphenylhydantoin in patients with epilepsy. Agreement between the unbound fraction in plasma and the concentration in the cerebrospinal fluid.' *Clin. Pharmac. Ther.* **13**, 196–200

47.   Mawer, G. E., Miller, N. E. and Turnberg, L. A. (1972). 'Metabolism of amylobarbitone in patients with chronic liver disease.' *Br. J. Pharmac.* **44**, 549–560

48.   Mitchell, J. R., Cavanaugh, J. H., Arias, L. and Oates, J. A. (1970). 'Guanethidine and related agents. III. Antagonism by drugs which inhibit the norepinephrine pump in man.' *J. clin. Invest.* **49**, 1596–1604

49.   Mitchell, J. R., Potter, W. Z., Jollow, D., Davis, D. C., Gillette, J. R. and Brodie, B. B. (1972). 'Acetaminophen-induced hepatic necrosis. I. Potentiation by inducers and protection by inhibitors of drug-metabolizing enzymes.' *Fedn Proc.* **31**, 539

50.   Mroczek, W. J., Leibel, B. A., Davidov, M. and Finnerty, F. A. (1971). 'The importance of the rapid administration of diazoxide in accelerated hypertension.' *New Engl. J. Med.* **285**, 603–606

51.   Neff, N. H. and Tozer, T. N. (1968). 'In vivo measurement of brain serotonin.' *Adv. Pharmacol.* **6A**, 97–109

52.   Odar-Cederlöf, I., Lunde, P. K. M. and Sjöqvist, F. (1970). 'Abnormal pharmacokinetics of diphenylhydantoin in a patient with uraemia.' *Lancet* **2**, 831–832

53.   O'Reilly, R. A. (1967). 'Studies on the coumarin anticoagulant drugs: interaction of human plasma albumin and warfarin sodium.' *J. clin. Invest.* **46**, 829–837

54.   Perl, W., Rackow, H., Salanitre, E., Wolf, G. L. and Epstein, R. M. (1965). 'Intertissue diffusion effect for inert fat-soluble gases.' *J. appl. Physiol.* **20**, 621–627

55.   Portmann, G. A., McChesney, E. W., Stander, H. and Moore, W. E. (1966). 'Pharmacokinetic model for nalidixic acid in man. II. Parameters for absorption, metabolism and elimination.' *J. pharm. Sci.* **55**, 72–78

56.   Price, H. L., Kovnat, P. J., Safer, J. N., Conner, E. H. and Price, M. L. (1960). 'The uptake of thiopental by body tissues and its relation to the duration of narcosis.' *Clin. Pharmac. Ther.* **1**, 16–22

57.   Rawlins, M. D. and Smith, S. E. (1972). 'Clinical pharmacology." In *Medical Progress 1971–72*, pp. 70–94. Ed. by Sir John Richardson. London: Butterworths

58.   Reidenberg, M. M., Odar-Cederlöf, I., Bahr, C. von, Borgå, O. and Sjöqvist, F. (1971). 'Protein binding of diphenylhydantoin

and desmethylimipramine in plasma from patients with poor renal function.' *New Engl. J. Med.* **285**, 264–267

59. Riegelman, S., Loo, J. C. K. and Rowland, M. (1968). 'Shortcomings in pharmacokinetic analysis by conceiving the body to exhibit properties of a single compartment.' *J. pharm. Sci.* **57**, 117–123

60. Rowland, M., Thomson, P. D., Guichard, A. and Melmon, K. L. (1971). 'Disposition kinetics of lidocaine in normal subjects.' *Ann. N.Y. Acad. Sci.* **179**, 383–398

61. Sellers, E. M. and Koch-Weser, J. (1969). 'Protein binding and vascular activity of diazoxide.' *New Engl. J. Med.* **281**, 1141–1145

62. Sellers, E. M. and Koch-Weser, J. (1970). 'Displacement of warfarin from human albumin by diazoxide, ethacrinic, mefenamic and nalidixic acids.' *Clin. Pharmac. Ther.* **11**, 524–529

63. Sellers, E. M. and Koch-Weser, J. (1971). 'Kinetics and clinical importance of displacement of warfarin from albumin by acidic drugs.' *Ann. N.Y. Acad. Sci.* **179**, 213–225

64. Shoeman, D. W. and Azarnow, D. L. (1972). 'The alteration of plasma proteins in uraemia as reflected by their activity to bind digitoxin and diphenylhydantoin.' *Pharmacology* **7**, 169–177

65. Silverman, W. A., Andersen, D. H., Blanc, W. A. and Crozier, D. N. (1956). 'A difference in mortality rate and incidence of kernicterus among premature infants alloted to two prophylactic antibacterial regimens.' *Pediatrics, Springfield* **18**, 614–625

66. Simpson, F. O. and Waal-Manning, H. J. (1971). 'Hypertension and depression: interrelated problems in therapy.' *Jl R. Coll. Physn. Lond.* **6**, 14–24

67. Skinner, C., Coull, D. C. and Johnston, A. W. (1969). 'Antagonism of the hypotensive action of bethanidine and debrisoquine by tricyclic antidepressants.' *Lancet* **2**, 564–566

68. Solomon, H. M. and Schrogie, J. J. (1967). 'The effect of phenyramidol on the metabolism of diphenylhydantoin.' *Clin. Pharmac. Ther.* **8**, 554–556

69. Solomon, H. M., Schrogie, J. J. and Williams, D. (1968). 'The displacement of phenylbutazone-^{14}C and warfarin-^{14}C from human albumin by various drugs and fatty acids.' *Biochem. Pharmac.* **17**, 143–151

70. Sönksen, P. H., Srivastava, M. C. and Tompkins, C. V. (1971). 'Antibiotic levels on continuous intravenous infusion.' *Lancet* **2**, 491

71. Sonnen, A. E. H. (1971). 'Misleading PBI.' *Lancet* **2**, 547

72. van der Kleijn, E. (1971). 'Pharmacokinetics of distribution and metabolism of ataractic drugs and an evaluation of the site of antianxiety activity.' *Ann. N.Y. Acad. Sci.* **179**, 115–125

73. Waddell, W. J. and Butler, T. C. (1957). 'The distribution and excretion of phenobarbital.' *J. clin. Invest.* **36**, 1217–1226

74. Wang, J. H. and Takemori, A. E. (1972). 'Studies on the transport of morphine into the cerebrospinal fluid of rabbits.' *J. Pharmac. exp. Ther.* **183**, 41–48

75. Wolff, J., Standaert, M. E. and Rall, J. E. (1961). 'Thyroxine displacement from serum proteins and depression of serum protein-bound iodine by certain drugs.' *J. clin. Invest.* **40**, 1373–1379

76. Wyers, P. J. H. and van Munster, P. J. J. (1961). 'The disappearance of Evans Blue dye from the blood in normal and nephrotic subjects.' *J. Lab. clin. Med.* **58**, 375–385

77. Zubrod, C. G., Kennedy, T. J. and Shannon, J. A. (1948). 'Studies on the chemotherapy of the human malarias. VIII. The physiological disposition of pamaquine.' *J. clin. Invest.* **27** (Suppl.), 114–120

CHAPTER 5

Drug Metabolism: General Principles

The majority of drugs used in man are non-polar, highly lipid-soluble compounds which cannot be excreted readily by the kidney because of back diffusion in the renal tubules. Calculations show that were it not for metabolism such compounds would be disposed of very slowly with a plasma half-life of some 24 days[9]. Furthermore, if the compound, like mepacrine or thiopentone, were reversibly sequestered in tissues, then its half-life would approach 100 years, which as Brodie[5] points out is longer than those of the doctor and patient combined. The processes of metabolism result in the formation of derivatives which are usually more polar, less lipid-soluble and therefore more readily excreted. In most cases the metabolites are less pharmacologically active than the parent compounds, although there are some exceptions to this generalization. Thus the first metabolites of imipramine (desipramine) and chloral hydrate (trichloroethanol) are highly active and probably responsible for most of the activity of the parent drugs. Similarly, the analgesic action of the newly introduced drug, benorylate, depends on its hydrolysis to yield the components aspirin and paracetamol. Drug toxicity may also be increased by metabolism. Thus the acetylated derivatives of many sulphonamides are less water-soluble than their parent compounds and are consequently more likely to precipitate in the renal tubule, causing haematuria, whilst epoxide derivatives of otherwise non-toxic aromatic substances such as bromobenzene are potent liver-necrotizing agents[6]

Pathways of drug metabolism

The pathways of drug metabolism are complex but they can conveniently be divided into two phases[46]. In phase I compounds undergo oxidation, reduction or hydrolysis. These processes expose or add functionally reactive groups which are then available for the synthetic (conjugating) mechanisms of phase II. These two metabolic stages are clearly seen in the metabolism of phenacetin, which is first dealkylated to form paracetamol (with its functionally reactive hydroxyl group) and subsequently conjugated with glucuronic acid:

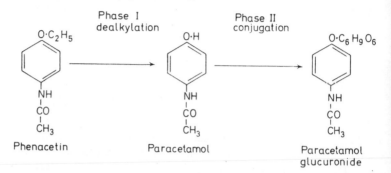

Drugs which already possess reactive groups are susceptible to conjugation without prior oxidation, reduction or hydrolysis. Thus morphine and chloramphenicol, which have hydroxyl groups, are metabolized to form glucuronides, and sulphonamides, which have amine groups, are acetylated. Phase I and phase II metabolic pathways and drugs which follow them are indicated in Table 5.1.

Hepatic drug metabolism

The majority of drugs are metabolized in the liver. The most frequently involved enzymes are those of the smooth-surfaced endoplasmic reticulum which separates on tissue homogenization and centrifugation into small particles, the microsomes. Microsomal enzymes, though small in number, are relatively non-specific in their affinity for different substrates and can each metabolize compounds of widely disparate structure. Many drugs, including opiates, phenothiazines, barbiturates, anticoagulants and hypoglycaemic agents, are oxidized by a mixed-function oxidase system. The over-all reaction brought about can be considered thus:

$$NADPH + drug + oxygen \longrightarrow NADP + oxidized\ drug + water$$

TABLE 5.1. Scheme of Drug Metabolic Pathways. Drug Examples Shown
in Parentheses

PHASE I

1. Oxidation

NADPH-dependent mixed function oxidases:

aromatic hydroxylation	(antipyrine)
aliphatic hydroxylation	(pentobarbitone)
deamination	(amphetamine)
N-dealkylation	(imipramine)
N-hydroxylation	(trimethylamine)
O-dealkylation	(codeine, phenacetin)
sulphoxidation	(chlorpromazine)
S-dealkylation	(6-methylthiopurine)
desulphuration	(thiopentone)
dehalogenation	(dicophane-DDS)
Dehydrogenation	(ethanol)
Oxidative deamination	(tyramine)

2. Reduction

Azoreduction	(Prontosil)
Nitroreduction	(chloramphenicol)
Carbonylreduction	(chloral hydrate)

3. Hydrolysis

De-esterification	(procaine, suxamethonium)
Deamidation	(procainamide)

PHASE II

4. Conjugation

Glucuronidation	(morphine)
Methylation:	
N-methylation	(noradrenaline)
S-methylation	(dimercaprol-BAL)
Acylation:	
acetylation	(sulphadimidine)
amino acids, e.g. glycine	(salicylate)
Mercapturic acid formation	(naphthalene)
Sulphate formation	(salicylamide)

Adapted from Gillette, 1967[18]

Reduced nicotinamide adenine diphosphate (NADPH) and oxygen are thus essential to the reaction. In addition, it requires the presence of a haem-containing protein which, because of its spectral characteristics when combined with carbon monoxide, is known as cytochrome P-450. This cytochrome exists in both oxidized and reduced states (see *Figure 5.1*). In the oxidized state (I) it combines with the drug to form a cytochrome P-450–drug complex (II) and this undergoes reduction by cytochrome P-450 reductase. The reduced cytochrome P-450–drug complex (III) then combines with oxygen (IV), following which the oxidized drug (V) is released and the cytochrome reverts to its oxidized state (I).

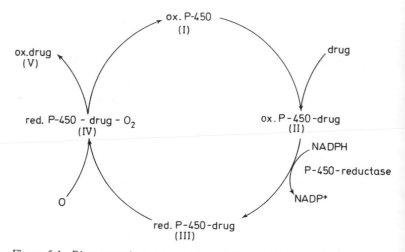

Figure 5.1. Diagrammatic representation of drug oxidation mediated by cytochrome P-450. The reduction of oxidized cytochrome P-450–drug complex (II) is brought about by cytochrome P-450 reductase either directly or through a carrier. The reductase is itself maintained in a reduced state by NADPH

Differences between individuals in the amount of cytochrome P-450 and cytochrome P-450 reductase would be expected to produce pronounced alterations in the rate at which any one drug is metabolized. Concentrations of cytochrome P-450 reductase in needle biopsy and post-mortem specimens of healthy human liver show about four- to sixfold differences between individuals[32, 35, 40], the values corresponding quite well to the rates of drug oxidation obtained *in vitro*. It seems likely that this degree of variability is sufficient to account for the differences in drug metabolism detected *in vivo*. Vesell and his colleagues[42], for example, quote figures for plasma half-lives of antipyrine (6.0–15.1 hours), phenylbutazone (1.2–7.3 days) and dicoumarol (7.0–74.0 hours), the ranges of which are roughly predictable. Another study on dicoumarol[39] and one on fenfluramine[10] show variability of a similar order.

Conjugation of a wide variety of drugs and drug metabolites with glucuronic acid also occurs within the liver microsomes, and is mediated by the enzyme glucuronyl transferase. The process does not occur directly but requires the activation of glucuronic acid by the synthesis of uridine diphosphate glucuronic acid (UDPGA) in the cytoplasm from glucose-1-phosphate and uridine diphosphate. Within the microsomes the reaction proceeds thus:

$$UDP-glucuronic\ acid\ +\ drug \longrightarrow drug-glucuronic\ acid\ +\ UDP$$

The activity of microsomal enzymes is one of the most important determinants of variability in drug response in man, the principal reason being that when drugs are given in repeated doses (as most are) the degree to which they accumulate is limited by the rate of their inactivation (see Chapter 2). Thus, on repeated administration to a patient with highly active enzymes, drugs susceptible to hepatic metabolism will accumulate to reach low steady-state levels, whereas in a patient with less active enzymes the same drugs will accumulate to reach much higher levels (see Chapter 2). The magnitude of the difference involved is well illustrated by the observations of Loeser[29], who found twelve-fold differences in steady-state plasma concentrations of phenytoin *(Figure 5.2.)*, and by those of Hammer and Sjöqvist[22], who found more than thirtyfold differences in steady-state plasma concentrations of desipramine in psychiatric patients *(Figure 5.3)*. In both instances the subjects received identical drug doses. Whether such extreme differences can be explained on the basis of differing concentrations of hepatic cytochrome P-450 and its reductase or whether other factors are involved is not known. As expected, alteration of the rate of drug metabolism in the individual patient inevitably alters its steady-state plasma concentration. This is well shown by the influence of treatment with phenobarbitone (an enzyme inducer – see Chapter 7) on the steady-state plasma concentration of desipramine[20] which is illustrated in *Figure 5.4*. Such differences must be of enormous therapeutic consequence (see Chapter 10).

When drugs are administered orally or by intraperitoneal injection they must first pass into the portal system and through the liver before reaching the systemic circulation. If the clearance of a drug by the liver is high, the amount that is actually available for distribution to the

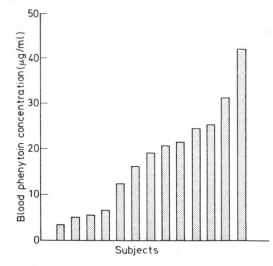

Figure 5.2. Steady-state plasma concentrations of phenytoin in 13 subjects following oral administration of phenytoin 400 mg daily for at least 14 days. (From Loeser, 1961[29])

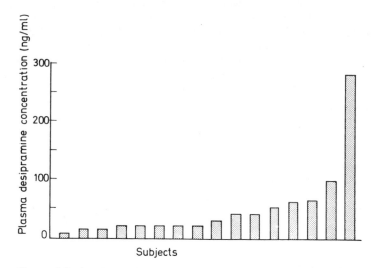

Figure 5.3. Steady-state plasma concentrations of desipramine in 16 subjects following oral administration of desipramine 25 mg three times daily for 10 days. (From Hammer and Sjöqvist, 1967[22])

various organs may be considerably less than the amount absorbed from the gastrointestinal tract. This so-called 'first-pass' effect[17] has been shown to influence the availability of salicylate, salicylamide, propranolol and nortriptyline. Furthermore, because of interindividual

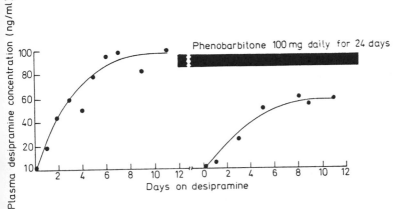

Figure 5.4. The effect of phenobarbitone administration on the plasma concentration of desipramine given 75 mg daily. The steady-state plasma concentration is halved when metabolism is accelerated by phenobarbitone. (From Hammer, Ideström and Sjöqvist, 1967[20])

differences in the capacity of the liver to metabolize drugs (see above) the first-pass effect can lead to differences in their systemic availability irrespective of their completeness of absorption. Thus the bioavailability of nortriptyline was found to vary from 55 to 70 per cent in three subjects in whom this was investigated[3]. The position with propranolol is complicated by the fact that although it undergoes oxidation at first-pass to 4-hydroxypropranolol when given by mouth but not when given intravenously[34], beta-blockade is greater than expected on the basis of plasma concentrations of the parent drug after oral dosage. The explanation appears to be that the 4-hydroxy derivative has pharmacological activity[11]. In view of the frequency with which the intraperitoneal route is used in experimental pharmacology on animals, it is interesting to reflect on the large number of compounds (good and bad) which may never have been considered for clinical use because of their destruction by the first-pass effect.

The factors which control the amount of drug-metabolizing ability in the liver microsomes are still the subject of investigation. There appear to be inherent control mechanisms which produce repression and removal of repression (known as derepression)[30] and it seems possible that these exert their effects by altering the rates of synthesis and destruction of the oxidizing and conjugating enzymes and of cytochrome P-450[19] and cytochrome P-450 reductase. In this method of control, both genetic and environmental influences are apparent. Many such aspects have been discussed in a recent symposium[41].

Drug metabolism in other sites

A small number of clinically useful drugs are metabolized in other tissues besides the liver. Thus levodopa is decarboxylated to form dopamine in the gastrointestinal tract and the kidney as well as in the liver by enzymes which are so active that only a small proportion of the drug is available to the brain. In the treatment of parkinsonism the effective dose of levodopa can be reduced about tenfold by the administration of the peripheral decarboxylase inhibitor methyldopa hydrazine[12]. Extrahepatic metabolism also affects many amines which are degraded by amine oxidases present in the intestine, the kidney, the lung and plasma. Plasma cholinesterase is responsible for inactivating suxamethonium, procaine and propanidid, and is subject to quantitative and qualitative variability (see Chapter 6).

Drug metabolism can occur both within the lumen of the gastrointestinal tract and in the intestinal wall. Peptidases of the intestinal secretions destroy orally administered polypeptide drugs and thus reduce their bioavailability by this route to zero. On the other hand, enzymes secreted into the intestinal lumen may also be responsible for hydrolysing drug conjugates which have been excreted via the bile. Thus morphine and chloramphenicol may be recycled and show further activity after reabsorption. Hydrolysis of drug conjugates is also performed by bacteria in the large intestine and such processes are responsible for the liberation of emodin, the active principle of the anthraquinone purgatives cascara and senna, and perhaps for the splitting of some cardiac glycosides. Bacterial drug metabolism is the subject of a recent review[37]. Both isoprenaline and chlorpromazine are extensively conjugated with sulphate during their passage through the intestinal wall. This process accounts for the fact that 10 mg isoprenaline administered orally has the same effect as 10 μg given intravenously[15].

Influence of age on drug metabolism

Inability to metabolize drugs may place the patient at risk of toxicity. This is particularly important in the very young and the very old.

Neonates have poor microsomal enzymes and cannot conjugate chlor-amphenicol[45], sulphonamides[16, 25], paracetamol[44] or mepro-bamate[47]. Conjugation of para-aminobenzoate is also reduced[43]. Hence the well known cyanosis (grey syndrome) which accompanies the use of chloramphenicol in young babies. It is also worth noting in this respect that chloramphenicol can cross the placental barrier and might therefore produce foetal toxicity in the pregnant mother.

Recent work suggests that some elderly patients also have defective enzyme activity as indicated by rather long antipyrine and phenylbuta-zone half-lives[33]. Limited ability to metabolize drugs is also crucial in the response to the anticonvulsant phenytoin and possibly also to salicylates[28]. The probable explanation is that at plasma concentra-tions reached clinically these compounds are metabolized at the maxi-mum rate possible and that consequently their elimination rate is limited by the amount of enzyme rather than the amount of drug. Rate-limited metabolism is discussed by Dayton and Perel[14]. The work of Kutt and his colleagues[26, 27] suggests that phenytoin toxicity (nystagmus, ataxia and mental changes) is linked to a low maximum rate of metabolism of this drug and that this defect may be familial in origin (see Chapter 6).

Tests of microsomal enzyme function

There is accumulating evidence reported here and in Chapters 6 and 7 that the individual rate of drug metabolism is an important deter-minant of clinical drug effect. On the basis of the kinetics discussed in Chapter 2, measurement of individual drug half-life or clearance should have predictive value for the clinical response. In a recent study of nortriptyline, Alexanderson[2] has confirmed that there is a very good correlation between single-dose clearance values and multiple-dose steady-state plasma concentrations, and it is known from other evi-dence that the latter are the clinical determinants. Unfortunately, measurements of nortriptyline and of many other drugs are time con-suming and (relatively) expensive. This makes the use of a prototype model drug (of easy and specific measurement) desirable.

A certain amount of evidence suggests that there is coincidence in man of the relative rates of metabolism of a wide variety of drugs which makes the use of a prototype justifiable. Thus, Hammer, Mårtens and Sjöqvist[21], measuring steady-state concentrations of desipramine and nortriptyline and half-lives of oxyphenbutazone, deduced a high cor-relation in the metabolism of these compounds. Single-dose half-lives of glutethimide and amylobarbitone have been shown to correlate[24] although neither correlated with half-lives of antipyrine, a drug which is frequently used as a prototype. Furthermore, a recent study by Smith and Rawlins[38] has indicated correlations of only a low order between plasma half-lives of antipyrine, phenylbutazone and warfarin. The correlation matrix is shown in Table 5.2. The interpretation of phenylbutazone half-life measurements is, however, complicated by the fact that the drug is both an inhibitor and an inducer of its own metabolism. Davies and Thorgeirsson[13] have found that after 5 days' administration, half-lives are sometimes shorter than after single doses.

TABLE 5.2. Correlation Coefficient Matrix for Single-dose Plasma Half-lives of Antipyrine, Phenylbutazone and Warfarin, 24-hour Excretion Rates of D-glucaric Acid and 6β-Hydroxycortisol and Serum Gamma-glutamyl Transpeptidase Activity in 16 Healthy Subjects

		r values					
		I	*II*	*III*	*IV*	*V*	*VI*
I	Antipyrine $T_{1/2}$	–	0.581[†]	0.384	0.112	0.033	–0.189
II	Phenylbutazone $T_{1/2}$	–	–	0.357	0.034	0.075	–0.082
III	Warfarin $T_{1/2}$	–	–	–	0.001	–0.283	–0.402
IV	D-glucaric acid excretion	–	–	–	–	0.140	–0.265
V	6β-Hydroxycortisol excretion	–	–	–	–	–	–0.171
VI	Serum gamma-glutamyl transpeptidase	–	–	–	–	–	–

[†]$p < 0.05$

They have also found that after 5 days, phenylbutazone half-lives and single-dose antipyrine half-lives correlate much better, possibly because at this stage neither inhibition nor induction is predominant. Furthermore, with phenylbutazone and with many other drugs metabolism is limited to a greater or lesser extent by sequestration of the drug by protein binding, tissue binding and storage in fat depots. It seems likely, therefore, that the use of a prototype is valid only if it is metabolized in the same pathway as that followed by the drug under investigation and if sequestration of the two is at least similar. On this basis, the lack of correlation found in the investigations quoted above reflects merely differences in these essential parameters and is hardly surprising.

Partly because of ease of determination, antipyrine[7, 31] and phenylbutazone[8] are most frequently used as prototypes for single-dose plasma half-life determinations.

Under conditions of marked enzyme induction when much more enzyme activity occurs in hepatic microsomes (see Chapter 7), activation of endogenous metabolic pathways has been shown to occur. Thus hydroxylation of cortisol increases, with the result that urinary 6β-hydroxycortisol excretion rises[4]. Similarly, activation of the glucuronidation pathway causes an increased urinary excretion of D-glucaric acid[1, 23], which is an end-product of D-glucuronic acid breakdown. There is also a recent finding[36] that with induction the level of plasma gamma-glutamyl transpeptidase rises, although whether this rise is a direct result of enzyme induction or a non-specific consequence of increased hepatic blood flow and increased cellular breakdown is not known. By implication, high urinary 6β-hydroxycortisol and D-glucaric acid excretion and high plasma gamma-glutamyl transpeptidase values can be taken to indicate the presence of enzyme induction and the likelihood that the individual will be relatively tolerant of drugs susceptible to hepatic metabolic inactivation. It would, of course, be convenient if such measurements could be used to predict rates of drug metabolism even in the absence of overt enzyme induction. It has been found, however, that in drug-free healthy subjects these measurements do not correlate with abilities to dispose of antipyrine, phenylbutazone and warfarin[38] (Table 5.2). It is therefore evident that they have no predictive value in the normal healthy state.

References

1. Aarts, E. M. (1965). 'Evidence for the function of D-glucaric acid as an indicator for drug induced enhanced metabolism through the glucuronic acid pathway in man.' *Biochem. Pharmac.* **14**, 359–363

2. Alexanderson, B. (1972). 'Pharmacokinetics of nortriptyline in man after single or multiple oral doses: the predictability of steady-state plasma concentrations from single-dose plasma-level data.' *Eur. J. clin. Pharmac.* **4**, 82–91

3. Alexanderson, B., Borgå, O. and Alvan, G. (1972). 'Studies on the availability of nortriptyline on oral administration.' *Eur. J. clin. Pharmac.* In press

4. Breckenridge, A., Orme, M.L'E., Thorgeirsson, S., Davies, D. S. and Brooks, R. V. (1971). 'Drug interactions with warfarin: studies with dichloralphenazone, chloral hydrate and phenazone (antipyrine).' *Clin. Sci.* **40**, 351–364

5.   Brodie, B. B. (1964). 'Distribution and fate of drugs; therapeutic implications.' In *Absorption and Distribution of Drugs*, pp. 199–251. Ed. by T. B. Binns. Edinburgh and London: Churchill Livingstone

6.   Brodie, B. B. (1972). 'Enzymatic activation of foreign compounds to more potent or more toxic derivatives.' *Abstr. Proc. 5th Int. Congr. Pharmacol.* p. 5. Basle: Karger

7.   Brodie, B. B., Axelrod, J., Soberman, R. and Levy, B. B. (1949). 'The estimation of antipyrine in biological materials.' *J. biol. Chem.* **179**, 25–29

8.   Burns, J. J., Rose, R. K., Chenkin, T., Goldman, A., Schulert, A. and Brodie, B. B. (1953). 'The physiological disposition of phenylbutazone (Butazolidin) in man and a method for its estimation in biological material.' *J. Pharmac. exp. Ther.* **109**, 346–357

9.   Butler, T. C. (1958). 'Termination of drug action by elimination of unchanged drug.' *Fedn Proc.* **17**, 1158–1162

10. Campbell, D. B. (1971). 'Plasma concentrations of fenfluramine and its metabolite norfenfluramine, after single and repeated oral administration.' *Br. J. Pharmac.* **43**, 465P–466P

11. Cleaveland, C. R. and Shand, D. G. (1972). 'Effect of route of administration on the relationship between β-adrenergic blockade and plasma propranolol level.' *Clin. Pharmac. Ther.* **13**, 181–185

12. Cotzias, G. C., Papavasiliou, P. S. and Gellene, R. (1969). 'Modification of parkinsonism – chronic treatment with L-dopa.' *New Engl. J. Med.* **280**, 337–345

13. Davies, D. S. and Thorgeirsson, S. S. (1971). 'Mechanism of hepatic drug oxidation and its relationship to individual differences in rates of oxidation in man.' *Ann. N.Y. Acad. Sci.* **179**, 411–420

14. Dayton, P. G. and Perel, J. M. (1971). 'Physiological and physicochemical bases of drug interactions in man.' *Ann. N.Y. Acad. Sci.* **179**, 67–87

15. Dollery, C. T., Davies, D. S. and Conolly, M. E. (1971). 'Differences in the metabolism of drugs depending upon their routes of administration.' *Ann. N.Y. Acad. Sci.* **179**, 108–114

16. Fiehter, E. G. and Curtis, J. A. (1955). 'Sulfonamide administration in newborn and premature infants.' *Am. J. Dis. Child.* **90**, 596–597

17. Gibaldi, M. (1971). 'Pharmacokinetic aspects of drug metabolism.' *Ann. N.Y. Acad. Sci.* **179**, 19–31

18. Gillette, J. R. (1967). 'Individually different responses to drugs according to age, sex and functional or pathological state.' In *Drug Responses in Man*, pp. 24–49. Ciba Foundation Symposium. Ed. by G. Wolstenholme and R. Porter. Edinburgh and London: Churchill Livingstone

19. Greim, H. and Remmer, H. (1969). 'Abbauhemmung und Synthesesteigerung bie der Vermehrung mikrosomaler Cytochrome durch Phenobarbital.' *Naunyn-Schmiedebergs Arch. exp. Path. Pharmak.* **264**, 238–239

20. Hammer, W., Ideström, C.-M. and Sjöqvist, F. (1967). 'Chemical control of antidepressant drug therapy.' In *Anti-Depressant Drugs*, Excerpta Medica Int. Congr. Series 122, pp. 301–310. Amsterdam: Excerpta Medica

21. Hammer, W., Mårtens, S. and Sjöqvist, F. (1969). 'A comparative study of the metabolism of desmethylimipramine, nortriptyline and oxyphenylbutazone in man.' *Clin. Pharmac. Ther.* **10**, 44–49

22. Hammer, W. and Sjöqvist, F. (1967). 'Plasma levels of monomethylated tricyclic antidepressants during treatment with imipramine-like compounds.' *Life Sci.* **6**, 1895–1903

23. Hunter, J., Maxwell, J. D., Carrella, M., Stewart, D. A. and Williams, R. (1971). 'Urinary D-glucaric-acid excretion as a test for hepatic enzyme induction in man.' *Lancet* **1**, 572–575

24. Kadar, D., Inaba, T., Endrenyi, L., Johnson, G. E. and Kalow, W. (1972). 'Drug metabolism in healthy subjects.' *Fedn Proc.* **31**, 537

25. Krauer, B., Spring. P. and Dettli, L. (1968). 'Zur Pharmakokinetik der Sulfonamide in ersten Lebensjahr.' *Pharmacologia Clin.* **1**, 47–53

26. Kutt, H., Winters, W., Kokenge, R. and McDowell, F. (1964). 'Diphenylhydantoin metabolism, blood levels and toxicity.' *Archs Neurol., Chicago* **11**, 642–648

27. Kutt, H., Wolk, M., Scherman, R. and McDowell, F. (1964). 'Insufficient parahydroxylation as a cause of diphenylhydantoin toxicity.' *Neurology, Minneap.* **14**, 542–548

28. Levy, G., Tsuchiya, T. and Amsel, L. P. (1972). 'Limited capacity for salicyl phenolic glucuronide formation and its effect on the kinetics of salicylate elimination in man.' *Clin. Pharmac. Ther.* **13**, 258–268

29. Loeser, E. W. (1961). 'Studies on the metabolism of diphenylhydantoin (Dilantin).' *Neurology, Minneap.* **11**, 424–429

30. Long, R. F. (1969). 'Induction of drug-metabolizing enzymes and cytochrome P-450.' *Biochem. J.* **115**, 26P

31. Mendelsohn, D. and Levin, N. W. (1960). 'A colorimetric micromethod for the estimation of antipyrine in plasma or serum.' *S. Afr. J. med. Sci.* **25**, 13–18

32. Nelson, E. B., Raj, P. P., Belfi, K. J. and Masters, B. S. S. (1971). 'Oxidative drug metabolism in human liver microsomes.' *J. Pharmac. exp. Ther.* **178**, 580–588

33. O'Malley, K., Crooks, J., Duke, E. and Stevenson, I. H. (1971). 'Effect of age and sex on human drug metabolism.' *Br. med. J.* **3**, 607–609

34. Paterson, J. W., Conolly, M. E. and Dollery, C. T. (1970). 'The pharmacodynamics and metabolism of propranolol in man.' *Pharmacologia Clin.* **2**, 127–133

35. Remmer, H., Schoene, B., Fleischmann, R. A. and Oldershausen, H. F.v. (1972). 'Drug metabolizing enzymes determined in needle biopsy material of human liver.' *Abstr. Proc. 5th Int. Congr. Pharmacol.,* p. 191. Basle: Karger

36. Rosalki, S. B., Tarlow, D. and Rau, D. (1971). 'Plasma gamma-glutamyl transpeptidase elevation in patients receiving enzyme-inducing drugs.' *Lancet* **2**, 376–377

37. Scheline, R. R. (1968). 'Drug metabolism by intestinal organisms.' *J. pharm. Sci.* **57**, 2021–2037

38. Smith, S. E. and Rawlins, M. D. (1973). 'Indicators of drug metabolising activity in man.' In preparation

39. Solomon, A. M. and Schrogie, J. J. (1967). 'The anticoagulant response to bishydroxycoumarin. 1. The role of individual variation.' *Clin. Pharmac. Ther.* **8**, 65–69

40. Thorgeirsson, S. S. and Davies, D. S. (1971). 'Kinetic studies of the N-demethylation of ethylmorphine by a cytochrome P-450-dependent enzyme system in human liver microsomes.' *Biochem. J.* **122**, 30P

41. Vesell, E. S. (Ed.) (1971). 'Drug metabolism in man.' *Ann. N.Y. Acad. Sci.* **179**, 1–773

42. Vesell, E. S., Passananti, G. T., Greene, F. E. and Page, J. G. (1971). 'Genetic control of drug levels and of the induction of drug-metabolizing enzymes in man: individual variability in the extent of allopurinol and nortriptyline inhibition of drug metabolism.' *Ann. N.Y. Acad. Sci.* **179**, 752–773

43. Vest, M. R. and Rossier, R. (1963). 'Detoxification in the newborn: the ability of the newborn infant to form conjugates with glucuronic acid, glycine, acetate and glutathione.' *Ann. N.Y. Acad. Sci.* **111**, 183–197

44. Vest, M. and Streiff, R. R. (1959). 'Studies on glucuronide formation in newborn infants and older children. Measurement of p-aminophenol glucuronide levels in the serum after an oral dose of acetanilid.' *Am. J. dis. Child.* **98**, 688–693

45. Weiss, C. F., Glazko, A. J. and Weston, J. K. (1960). 'Chloramphenicol in the newborn infant: a physiological explanation of its toxicity when given in excessive dose.' *New Engl. J. Med.* **262**, 787–794

46. Williams, R. T. (1967). 'Comparative patterns of drug metabolism.' *Fedn Proc.* **26**, 1029–1039

47. Yu, W. L. and Aldrich, R. A. (1960). 'The glucuronyl transferase system in the newborn infant.' *Pediat. Clins N. Am.* **7**, 381–396

CHAPTER 6

Drug Metabolism: Genetic Factors

The rate and manner in which the individual metabolizes drugs is partly determined by his or her inheritance. The genes involved can conveniently be divided into two types. Genes of large effect are those which, on their own, determine a recognizable character in the individual. Their recognition enables one to distinguish different phenotypes in a population and therefore the existence of a polymorphism. Such genes influence drug metabolism by determining the amount and the nature of particular enzymes, although by comparison with the number of enzyme variants which probably exist[16] the number which are of known pharmacological interest or importance is rather small. Some of these enzyme variants are exceedingly rare and their presence may be said to expose the individual to a drug idiosyncrasy. The frequency with which a recognizably different enzyme reaction is found depends on the particular gene frequency in the population. Such gene frequencies are sometimes found to differ among different population groups and to lead to an uneven world distribution, although in many cases the selective forces responsible for their maintenance cannot be identified. One consequence of uneven world distribution is that the results of drug treatments must be expected to vary widely in different populations. It is common clinical experience to read of different success rates in clinical drug trials from different parts of the world. In some instances the possible part played by genetic polymorphisms would be worth investigation.

By contrast, genes of small effect do not produce recognizable characters on their own but, acting together, a large number of them contribute to individual deviation in a normally distributed population.

Thus, just as some people are taller or shorter than others, so individuals can metabolize drugs at faster or slower rates. The heritable influences are said to be polygenic. To the extent that the presence of genes of large effect does not exclude the presence of genes of small effect, both types must coexist. Indeed, the difference between them is merely one of recognition.

This chapter concerns only genetic influences on the metabolism of drugs. Reactions to drug administration are also affected by genes which influence tissue responses. For these the reader is referred to Chapter 9.

Genes of large effect

Hepatic drug acetylation

There is a wide variability in the extent to which individuals inactivate isoniazid by acetylation[5], much of the variability being genetic in origin[4]. Evans, Manley and McKusick[11] demonstrated that a

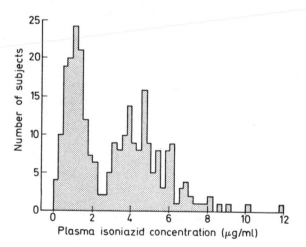

Figure 6.1. Plasma isoniazid concentrations in 483 subjects 6 hours after oral isoniazid 9.8 mg/kg. Polymorphism for acetylation causes a bimodal distribution in the population. (From Evans, Manley and McKusick, 1960[11])

polymorphism exists and that rapid inactivation is inherited as a dominant character which determines the presence of large amounts of the acetyltransferase concerned. Plasma concentrations which follow a single dose of isoniazid are illustrated in *Figure 6.1*. Their bimodal distribution contrasts markedly with the unimodal distribution of concentrations that follows the administration of salicylate *(Figure 6.2)* which is not influenced by a metabolic polymorphism. One consequence of the isoniazid polymorphism is that peripheral neuropathy as

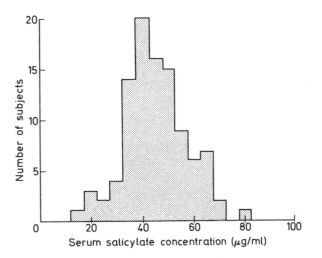

Figure 6.2. Serum salicylate concentrations in 100 subjects 3 hours after oral sodium salicylate 35 mg/kg. The values are approximately normally distributed. (From Evans and Clarke, 1961 [9])

a complication of isoniazid therapy for tuberculosis is more likely to occur in slow inactivators. Devadatta and his colleagues[8] found 17 cases among 83 slow inactivators (20 per cent) but only 2 cases among 60 rapid inactivators (3 per cent) treated with the drug. Furthermore, on widely spaced dose regimens, slow inactivators show somewhat better treatment responses[28] (Table 6.1). Both consequences arise from the persistence of higher plasma concentrations of the drug in the slow inactivators.

The acetylation polymorphism affects the metabolism of other drugs, too. Evans and White[12] demonstrated a coincidence of acetylation between isoniazid and sulphadimidine *in vivo* and also with hydrallazine *in vitro*. Among hypertensive subjects, slow inactivators have been found to require smaller doses of hydrallazine for blood pressure control[38] and they more commonly show toxic signs and develop antinuclear antibodies with this drug[24]. One might also expect greater development of antinuclear antibodies with isoniazid

TABLE 6.1. Tuberculosis Chemotherapy: Comparison of Twice-weekly and Once-weekly Treatment with Isoniazid 15 mg/kg plus Streptomycin. Figures are the numbers of patients with bacteriologically negative (and positive) sputum at 10, 11 and 12 months. On both treatment regimens, cure rates are higher among slow acetylators of isoniazid

Regimen	Slow acetylators of isoniazid	Rapid acetylators of isoniazid	χ^2	P
Twice weekly				
Quiescent	60	26		
Not quiescent	3	7	6.27	<0.01
All	63	33		
Once weekly				
Quiescent	29	20		
Not quiescent	9	19	5.22	<0.01
All	38	39		

From Tuberculosis Chemotherapy Centre, Madras, 1970[28]

therapy and consequent more frequent production of lupus erythematosus in the same group[1]. The same polymorphism affects the metabolism of phenelzine and slow inactivators treated with this drug appear to be more susceptible to its unwanted side-effects[10]. The metabolism of sulphamethoxypyridazine[35] and dapsone[14] are similarly influenced.

Slow inactivators are also more susceptible to drug interactions. Brennan and his colleagues[6] reported that toxicity to phenytoin with concurrent isoniazid in tuberculous patients was limited to slow inactivators, again presumably due to the persistent high plasma concentrations of the latter drug. The nature of the interaction is, however, obscure because different enzyme systems are involved, phenytoin being metabolized largely by hydroxylation.

The gene responsible for rapid inactivation is thought to have a mongoloid origin because its population frequency is greatest among Eskimos and Japanese and lowest among some Mediterranean Jews[22]. The expected differences in efficacy and toxicity of isoniazid do not appear to have been reported.

Plasma cholinesterase

In the great majority of patients the neuromuscular blocker suxamethonium has a duration of action of only a few minutes because the drug is rapidly metabolized by plasma cholinesterase (butyrylcholinesterase, pseudocholinesterase). In rare individuals suxamethonium induces neuromuscular blockade of 2–3 hours' duration instead of the usual few minutes[15] because the drug is not metabolized in the usual way. In such individuals the enzyme exists in a variant form which cannot hydrolyse this substrate and which also shows some other differences in its response to enzyme inhibitors. It is now known that many variant forms exist and that they are determined by genes of large effect. All these genes (Table 6.2) are uncommon and phenotypes who lack any enzyme capable of hydrolysing suxamethonium are very rare.

TABLE 6.2. Variants of Plasma Butyrylcholinesterase (Pseudocholinesterase)

Locus	Gene	Enzyme variant	Frequency of homozygotes
First	E_1^u	Usual	94%
	E_1^a	Atypical, dibucaine-resistant*	1 in 2,500
	E_1^f	Fluoride-resistant†	Very rare
	E_1^s	None (silent gene)*	Very rare
Second	E_2^-	c_5 electrophoretic bend absent	90%
	E_2^+	c_5 electrophoretic bend present	10%
Unknown	E^{Cl}	(Incompletely resolved ‡ chloride sensitivity)	Unknown
	E_{Cyn}	High activity §	Very rare

Data from Harris, 1964[15]; Simpson and Kalow, 1966[26]; Whittaker, 1968[37]

*Suxamethonium-sensitive
†Suxamethonium-partial sensitivity
‡Some varieties suxamethonium-sensitive
§Suxamethonium-resistant

The commonest of these are homozygotes for the the atypical enzyme ($E_1^a E_1^a$) but these are found with a frequency of only 1 in 2,500 in the population[17]. Heterozygotes ($E_1^u E_1^a$) who possess both the usual and the atypical enzymes make up about 4 per cent of the population; they can be distinguished only by *in vitro* tests[21]. Their clinical response to suxamethonium is normal.

Phenotype studies of patients showing prolonged apnoea following suxamethonium do not always reveal recognizable abnormalities. In some cases this can be accounted for by rather low plasma cholin-esterase values consequent upon malnutrition or liver disease, and in others excess cerebral depression by anaesthetic agents or body cooling may be responsible. Further cases still remain, however, when these causes are excluded. In a study of 104 patients showing suxametho-nium apnoea, Simpson and Kalow[26] surprisingly found 39 to be of the $E_1^u E_1^u$ phenotype. It is possible that these individuals may have an enzyme of a particular chloride sensitivity (E^{Cl}) more recently identi-fied by Whittaker[36] amongst a similar group of patients.

By contrast, atypical resistance to suxamethonium has also been described[23] in a family and shown to be due to the presence of an abnormally active form of butyrylcholinesterase, denoted $E_{Cynthiana}$, which is inherited as a dominant trait. It is conceivable that this is due to a variant on the second locus, at least one form of which, E_2^+, confers added activity to the enzyme.

Little is known of the distribution of these genes in different popula-tions, but Kalow and Gunn[18] found 4 atypical homozygotes among 2,442 patients of a mental hospital and Johnson and Lal (unpublished observations) found 3 among 1,032 patients and staff of a general hospital in Burma. More recently, a much higher incidence of the atypical enzyme has been reported among leprosy patients in South India[27]. These frequencies are significantly higher than those usually reported for healthy Caucasian populations. It is therefore possible that the incidence of suxamethonium apnoea may vary among different patient groups.

Hepatic dealkylation

The occurrence of marked methaemoglobinaemia following drug administration suggests that the individual cannot reduce this substance at a normal rate (see Chapter 9). A single case precipitated by phen-acetin has, however, been shown to be associated with partial failure of de-ethylation of the drug to form paracetamol with consequent accumulation of other metabolites[25]. The finding that a sister of the propositus had the same defect indicated an inherited defect caused by presence or absence of a gene of large effect. The chief objection is that phenacetin de-ethylation is catalysed by the ordinary microsomal mixed-function oxidases which are probably under polygenic control (see below). The family concerned may have microsomal enzymes which lack widespread metabolizing ability.

Similar factors may account for the apparent familial origin of phenytoin toxicity (Chapter 5) reported by Kutt and his colleagues[19, 20]. This condition arises in individuals who have a low maximum rate of phenytoin metabolism, as a result of which drug accumulation occurs yielding abnormally high plasma concentrations.

Genes of small effect

The rate of metabolism of most drugs appears to be genetically influenced by polygenic control. This is apparent from a number of studies on identical and fraternal twins, involving measurements of half-lives or steady-state concentrations of different drugs. Thus identical but not fraternal twins show very close agreement in their handling of phenylbutazone[30], as illustrated in *Figure 6.3,* and of dicoumarol[31], antipyrine[32], ethanol[33], halothane[7] and nortriptyline[2]. Similar findings have been reported with isoniazid[4], metabolism of which is now known to be determined by a gene of large effect (see above).

Although these results indicate that inheritance is a determinant of drug metabolism, the degree to which it is responsible for the variability in the population is uncertain. Indeed, because environmental influences differ from one population to another, it is to be expected that the apparent heritability must also differ somewhat. Estimates of heritability derived from twin studies, such as those quoted above, are beset by methodological difficulties of data analysis[29], with the result that different methods yield widely discrepant estimates. Furthermore, one of the methods advocated[13] requires a comparison of two regression coefficients which involves large errors[36]. With this in mind, the calculated values for heritability yielded by three different methods shown in Table 6.3 provide at best only a rough indication and at worst little help at all. The values given for heritability of phenylbutazone metabolism are higher than the more reliable estimate of 0.65 yielded by the family study of Whittaker and Evans[36]. This latter estimate, however, must also be accepted with caution because although all the subjects were given phenobarbitone as an enzyme-inducing agent (Chapter 7) for 3 days to negate the possible influence of environmental inducers, it is doubtful if this period is long enough to produce complete induction in all subjects. The true value may therefore be slightly higher.

The implication of the twin and family studies is that the quantity of rate-limiting enzyme in the liver microsomes is genetically influenced and it is interesting in this respect that a family study of plasma butyrylcholinesterase has shown similar findings[34]. There is also support for the polygenic nature of the influence over nortriptyline metabolism. As shown by Åsberg, Evans and Sjöqvist[3], relatives of propositi who develop high steady-state plasma levels themselves

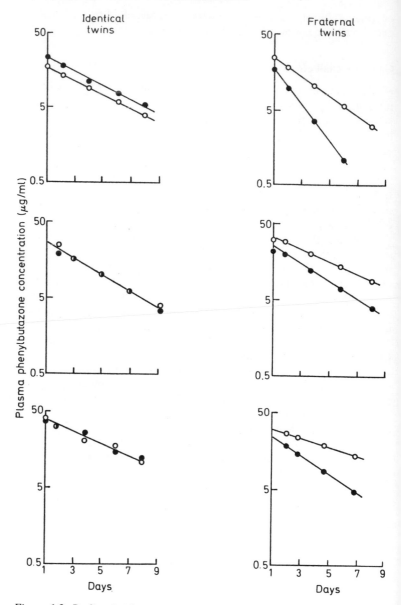

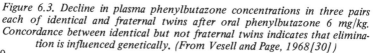

Figure 6.3. Decline in plasma phenylbutazone concentrations in three pairs each of identical and fraternal twins after oral phenylbutazone 6 mg/kg. Concordance between identical but not fraternal twins indicates that elimination is influenced genetically. (From Vesell and Page, 1968[30])

TABLE 6.3. Heritability of Variations in Drug Metabolism by Twin Subjects using Different Methods of Data Analysis

Drug	Heritability			Reference
	$\dfrac{V_F - V_I}{V_F}$	$\dfrac{r_I - r_F}{1 - r_F}$	$2(r_I - r_F)$	
Antipyrine	0.98	0.72	0.76	[32]
Dicoumarol	0.97	0.56	0.38	[31]
Ethanol	0.98	0.71	0.88	[33]
Halothane	0.88	0.25	0.32	[7]
Nortriptyline	–	–	0.81	[2]
Phenylbutazone	0.99	0.75	1.00	[30]
Plasma butyryl cholinesterase activity	0.60	0.65	0.67	[34]

Partly from Vesell, 1972 [29]

V_I and V_F = intrapair variances of identical and fraternal twins

r_I and r_F = intrapair correlation coefficients of identical and fraternal twins

develop steady-state levels which are high but normally distributed. The existence of a polymorphism is thereby excluded because such would have produced a bimodal or a trimodal distribution.

References

1. Alarcón-Segovia, D. (1969). 'Drug-induced lupus syndromes.' Mayo Clin. Proc. 44, 664–681
2. Alexanderson, B., Evans, D. A. P. and Sjöqvist, F. (1969). 'Steady-state plasma levels of nortriptyline in twins: influence of genetic factors and drug therapy.' Br. med. J. 4, 764–768
3. Åsberg, M., Evans, D. A. P. and Sjöqvist, F. (1971). 'Genetic control of nortriptyline kinetics in man – a study of relatives of propositi with high plasma concentration.' Chem.-Biol. Interactions 3. 238–240
4. Bönicke, R. and Lisboa, B. P. (1957). 'Über die Erbbedingtheit der intraindividuellen Konstanz der Isoniazidausscheidung beim Menschen (Untersuchungen an eineiigen und zweieiigen Zwillingen).' Naturwissenschaften 44, 314

81

5. Bönicke, R. and Reif, W. (1953). 'Enzymatische Inaktivierung von Isonicotinsäurehydrazid im menschlichen und tierischen Organismus.' *Naunyn-Schmiedebergs Arch. exp. Path. Pharmak.* **220**, 321–333

6. Brennan, R. W., Deheyia, H., Kutt, H. and McDowell, F. (1968). 'Diphenylhydantoin intoxication attendant to slow inactivation of isoniazid.' *Neurology, Minneap.* **18**, 283

7. Cascorbi, H. F., Vesell, E. S., Blake, D. A. and Helrich, M. (1971). 'Genetic and environmental influence on halothane metabolism in twins.' *Clin. Pharmac. Ther.* **12**, 50–55

8. Devadatta, S., Gangadharam, P. R. J., Andrews, R. H., Fox, W., Ramakrishnan, C. V., Selkon, J. B. and Velu, S. (1960). 'Peripheral neuritis due to isoniazid.' *Bull. Wld Hlth Org.* **23**, 587–598

9. Evans, D. A. P. and Clarke, C. A. (1961). 'Pharmacogenetics.' *Br. med. Bull.* **17**, 234–240

10. Evans, D. A. P., Davison, K. and Pratt, R. T. C. (1965). 'The influence of acetylator phenotype on the effects of treating depression with phenelzine.' *Clin. Pharmac. Ther.* **6**, 430–435

11. Evans, D. A. P., Manley, K. A. and McKusick, V. A. (1960). 'Genetic control of isoniazid metabolism in man.' *Br. med. J.* **2**, 485–491

12. Evans, D. A. P. and White, T. A. (1964). 'Human acetylation polymorphism.' *J. Lab. clin. Med.* **63**, 387–403

13. Falconer, D. A. (1960). *Introduction to Quantitative Genetics.* Edinburgh: Oliver and Boyd

14. Gelber, R., Peters, J. H., Gordon, G. R., Glazko, A. J. and Levy, L. (1971). 'The polymorphic acetylation of dapsone in man.' *Clin. Pharmac. Ther.* **12**, 225–238

15. Harris, H. (1964). 'Enzymes and drug sensitivity. The genetics of serum cholinesterase deficiency in relation to suxamethonium apnoea.' *Proc. R. Soc. Med.* **57**, 503–506

16. Harris, H., Hopkinson, D. A. and Luffman, J. (1968). 'Enzyme diversity in human populations.' *Ann. N.Y. Acad. Sci.* **151**, 232–242

17. Kalow, W. and Genest, K. (1957). 'A method for the detection of atypical forms of human serum cholinesterase. Determination of dibucaine numbers.' *Can. J. Biochem. Physiol.* **35**, 339–346

18. Kalow, W. and Gunn, D. R. (1959). 'Some statistical data on atypical cholinesterase of human serum.' *Ann. hum. Genet.* **23**, 239–250

19. Kutt, H., Winters, W., Kokenge, R. and McDowell, F. (1964). 'Diphenylhydantoin metabolism, blood levels, and toxicity.' *Archs Neurol.., Chicago* **11**, 642–648

20. Kutt, H., Wolk, M., Scherman, R. and McDowell, F. (1964). 'Insufficient parahydroxylation as a cause of diphenylhydantoin toxicity.' *Neurology, Minneap.* **14**, 542–548

21. Liddell, J., Lehmann, H., Davies, D. and Sharih, A. (1962). 'Physical separation of pseudocholinesterase variants in human serum.' *Lancet* 1, 463–464

22. Motulsky, A. G. (1964). 'Pharmacogenetics.' *Prog. med. Genet.* 3, 49–74

23. Neitlich, H. W. (1966). 'Increased plasma cholinesterase activity and succinylcholine resistance: a genetic variant.' *J. clin. Invest.* 45, 380–387

24. Perry, H. M., Sakamoto, A. and Tan, E. M. (1967). 'Relationship of acetylating enzyme to hydralazine toxicity.' *J. Lab. clin. Med.* 70, 1020–1021

25. Shahidi, N. T. (1967). 'Acetophenetidin sensivity.' *Am. J. Dis. Child.* 113, 81–82

26. Simpson, N. E. and Kalow, W. (1966). 'Pharmacology and biological variation.' *Ann. N.Y. Acad. Sci.* 134, 864–872

27. Thomas, M. and Job, C. K. (1972). 'Serum atypical pseudocholinesterase and genetic factors in leprosy.' *Br. med. J.* 3, 390–391

28. Tuberculosis Chemotherapy Centre, Madras (1970). 'A controlled comparison of a twice-weekly and three once-weekly regimens in the initial treatment of pulmonary tuberculosis.' *Bull. Wld Hlth Org.* 43, 143–206

29. Vesell, E. S. (1972). 'Introduction: genetic and environmental factors affecting drug response in man.' *Fedn Proc.* 31, 1253–1269

30. Vesell, E. S. and Page, J. G. (1968). 'Genetic control of drug levels in man: phenylbutazone.' *Science, N.Y.* 159, 1479–1480

31. Vesell, E. S. and Page, J. G. (1968). 'Genetic control of dicoumarol levels in man.' *J. clin. Invest.* 47, 2657–2663

32. Vesell, E. S. and Page, J. G. (1968). 'Genetic control of drug levels in man: antipyrine.' *Science, N.Y.* 161, 72–73

33. Vesell, E. S., Page, J. G. and Passananti, G. T. (1971). 'Genetic and environmental factors affecting ethanol metabolism in man.' *Clin. Pharmac. Ther.* 12, 192–201

34. Wetstone, H. J., Honeyman, M. S. and McComb, R. B. (1965). 'Genetic control of the quantitative activity of a serum enzyme in man.' *J. Am. med. Ass.* 192, 1007–1009

35. White, T. A. and Evans, D. A. P. (1968). 'The acetylation of sulphamethazine and sulphamethoxypyridazine by human subjects.' *Clin. Pharmac. Ther.* 9, 80–88

36. Whittaker, J. A. and Evans, D. A. P. (1970). 'Genetic control of phenylbutazone metabolism in man.' *Br. med. J.* 4, 323–328

37. Whittaker, M. (1968). 'An additional pseudocholinesterase phenotype occurring in suxamethonium apnoea.' *Br. J. Anaesth.* 40, 579–582

38. Zacest, R. and Koch-Weser, J. (1972). 'Relation of hydralazine plasma concentration to dosage and hypotensive action.' *Clin. Pharmac. Ther.* 13, 420–425

CHAPTER 7

Drug Metabolism:
Environmental Influences

The rate of drug metabolism *in vivo* is influenced by exposure to a wide variety of foreign chemical compounds and by disease. Such environmental factors affect drug metabolism by either increasing or decreasing enzyme activity.

Enzyme induction

Microsomal drug metabolism can be accelerated by a large number of different substances by a process known as enzyme induction. It is a complex process associated with a rise in liver weight, proliferation of the endoplasmic reticulum, increase in microsomal protein, a rise in cytochrome P-450 content and increased cytochrome P-450 reductase activity. Evidence from animal experiments indicates that the increases in cytochrome P-450 and its reductase are due to accelerated synthesis. There appears to be a coincident increase in hepatic blood flow and activation of some endogenous substrate metabolizing pathways. Thus, as discussed in Chapter 5, there is an increase in hydroxylation of cortisol to form 6β-hydroxycortisol[14] and increased D-glucuronic acid metabolism to form D-glucaric acid[51] and probably xylulose as well. In addition, serum levels of gamma-glutamyl transpeptidase rise[96], suggesting that there is a generalized increase in hepatic tissue turnover. Work on animals has revealed inducing effects of an enormous range of compounds which include drugs, hormones, aromatic hydrocarbons, insecticides, herbicides, food additives, dyes and carcinogens. Lists of these and a lengthy discussion of the importance of enzyme induction are contained in a review by Conney[20]. The mechanism whereby enzyme activity increases is not fully understood. It may involve derepression of enzyme synthesis and slowed breakdown of cytochrome P-450[67] and there is some evidence from animal work that this cytochrome has different properties according to the type of inducer used. At the chemical level, inducers such as barbiturates and collidines show a remarkable fit as false components in the haem template[41]. This is illustrated in *Figure 7.1*. If haem is a physiological

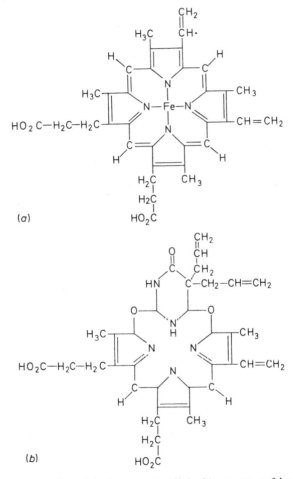

Figure 7.1. (a) Haem. (b) Allobarbitone as a false component on the haem template. Such a complex may not function as a corepressor of microsomal enzyme formulation, allowing induction (derepression) to occur. (From Granick, 1966[41])

corepressor which acts against enzyme formation, as seems likely, incorporation of such a false component would necessarily produce derepression and a consequent increase in enzyme formation. Different inducers might be expected to influence different repressors.

Induction and inheritance

The suggestion has been made that the degree of induction of the individual's microsomal enzymes in response to an inducing agent is determined genetically. Thus Vesell and Page[119] found agreement among four pairs of identical twins (but not among four pairs of fraternal twins) in the extent to which their antipyrine half-lives were shortened by phenobarbitone administration. The interpretation of this finding is, however, complicated by the fact that the degree of shortening achieved is strongly dependent on the initial half-life value. Those subjects with the longest half-lives showed the greatest degree of shortening, a finding which confirms other workers' observations[131] that the effect of an enzyme inducer is greatest in those subjects who have the poorest enzyme activity to start with. There may be two reasons for this. First, many enzyme inducers are themselves metabolized. By implication, therefore, the inducer persists in the circulation and in the liver for a shorter time in those individuals who metabolize it faster, thus minimizing its actions on the liver as elsewhere. Secondly, it seems likely that many individuals are already under the influence of unidentified inducing substances such as hydrocarbons and benzpyrenes in their environment, so that their response to inducing drugs is necessarily less. The work of Whittaker and Evans[131] on phenylbutazone metabolism is consistent with this hypothesis, for they found that there was a significant correlation between unrelated spouses in the half-life of this drug.

It is therefore uncertain whether induction as such is under genetic control or not. Analysis of the twin data excluding the influences discussed above leaves intrapair correlations (see Chapter 6) higher in identical ($r_I = 1.00$) than in fraternal ($r_F = 0.68$) twins, a finding which supports the original contention. With such small numbers, however, the errors inherent in the method do not allow a reliable estimate of heritability to be made.

Induction by drugs

Although hundreds of compounds have been shown to be effective enzyme inducers in animals, only a handful of these have been studied in man. In many cases animal experiments have involved the use of drugs in doses well outside any possible clinical range, suggesting that many of the positive findings may be irrelevant to the clinical situation. Thus chlordiazepoxide has been shown to induce enzymes in rats[49] but appears not to do so in man[95] or to have only a slight effect[8]. Similarly, the aldosterone antagonist, spironolactone, is an inducer in mice[38] although its influence at clinical doses on antipyrine metabolism in man is inconstant[114]. Furthermore, in man, apparent inducing agents do not necessarily influence all enzyme substrates in the same manner. Thus a recently reported hypolipidaemic agent, halofenate, which is related to clofibrate is said to shorten antipyrine and dicoumarol half-lives but lengthen that of warfarin[121]. It is therefore unwise to generalize about the effects of inducers in particular situations until they have been investigated. A list of substances known to cause enzyme induction in man is given in Table 7.1.

TABLE 7.1. Drugs and Other Substances Known to Cause Microsomal Enzyme Induction in Man

Barbiturates	Amylobarbitone, barbitone, cyclobarbitone, hexobarbitone, phenobarbitone, quinalbarbitone
Non-barbiturate hypnotics and tranquillizers	Chloral hydrate, chlordiazepoxide*, dichloralphenazone, glutethimide, meprobamate
Analgesics	Antipyrine, phenylbutazone
Chlorinated insecticides	Endrin, dicophane (DDT), gamma-benzene hexachloride (lindane)
Others	Carbamazepine, ethanol, griseofulvin, halofenate*, phenytoin, spironolactone*, cigarette smoking

*Drugs producing only slight or irregular induction

Most reports on enzyme induction in the clinical situation have been concerned with the effects of barbiturates, which can probably accelerate microsomal enzyme activity three or four times. The longer-acting barbiturates such as phenobarbitone have the most powerful inducing action, perhaps partly because they persist in the tissues for longer periods. Judging from animal experiments, however, other factors are involved, too. Amylobarbitone, for example, is never as effective an inducer as phenobarbitone even with repeated very high doses[7]. The greater efficacy of phenobarbitone is therefore not fully understood. The assumption is often made that barbiturate tolerance is largely the result of enzyme induction. This appears not to have been investigated, however, and the assumption may be unwarranted. Barbiturate tolerance in animals can occur in the absence of induction[33] and must presumably result from adaptive changes in the brain. The same may be true in man.

Hypnotic−anticoagulant interactions

Enzyme induction by barbiturates is of great importance in patients on anticoagulant therapy with the coumarin type of drug, largely because dosage control is so critical. The barbiturate accelerates metabolism of the anticoagulant and thus reduces both steady-state plasma

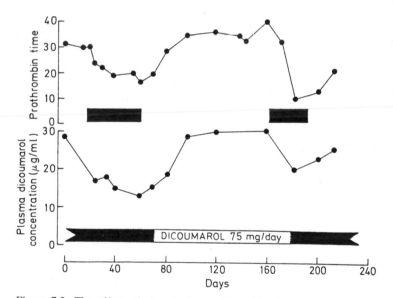

Figure 7.2. The effect of phenobarbitone 60 mg/day (upper solid bars) on steady-state plasma dicoumarol concentrations and prothrombin time in a patient receiving dicoumarol 75 mg/day. (From Burns and Conney, 1965[13])

concentrations and the prothrombin response[13, 23, 27, 39, 94]. The same is true of treatment with dichloralphenazone and antipyrine (phenazone)[8, 9], carbamazepine[47], griseofulvin[16] and probably any of the other drugs listed in Table 7.1. The effects of phenobarbitone, amylobarbitone and dichloralphenazone administration on anticoagulant therapy are illustrated in *Figures 7.2, 7.3 and 7.4.* Chloral hydrate, though possibly a weak enzyme inducer as indicated by its effect on dicoumarol metabolism[24], actually increases the anticoagulant effect of warfarin[105], probably because the trichloroacetic acid formed as a metabolite of the chloral displaces the anticoagulant from its plasma-protein-binding site[9] (see Chapter 4). Indeed, its apparent accelerating effect on anticoagulant metabolism may also be a consequence of this displacement.

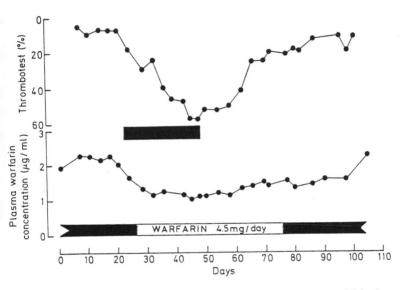

Figure 7.3. The effect of amylobarbitone 200 mg nightly (upper solid bar) on steady-state plasma warfarin concentrations and thrombotest activity in a patient receiving warfarin 4.5 mg/day. (From Breckenridge and Orme, 1971[8])

Dangerous interaction may thus occur if a patient takes an inducing agent while anticoagulant therapy is not being monitored or monitored only rarely; the treatment may become inadequate. Conversely, stopping treatment with the inducing agent may lead to excessive anticoagulation and consequent haemorrhage. Such an episode can occur at any time up to three weeks, or more in exceptional circumstances, after stopping treatment with the inducer, the delay being determined by the turnover rate of the microsomal enzymes involved. We have a strong impression that anticoagulant requirements were known for many years to be higher in hospitalized than in out-patients. In retrospect it is easy to see the reason for this, namely the consumption of hypnotic drugs by patients while in hospital and the cessation after they went home.

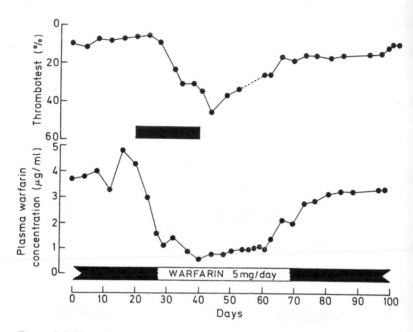

Figure 7.4. The effect of dichloralphenazone 1,300 mg nightly (upper solid bar) on steady-state plasma warfarin concentrations and thrombotest activity in a patient receiving warfarin 5 mg/day. (From Breckenridge and Orme, 1971[8])

Other drug interactions

Barbiturates accelerate metabolism and lower steady-state plasma concentrations of many other drugs such as tricyclic antidepressants[2, 43] *(Figure 5.3)*, griseofulvin[15], phenytoin[60, 75] and dicophane[26, 125]. Jelliffe and Blankenhorn[55] have reported the interesting finding that phenobarbitone accelerates the conversion of digitoxin to digoxin. It may also accelerate the metabolism of exogenous corticosteroids with consequent symptomatic deterioration in prednisone-dependent asthmatic patients[12]. Phenobarbitone treatment has also been used for its inducing action in neonatal and adult unconjugated hyperbilirubinaemia[70, 116, 130]. Dicophane has been used for the same purpose[115] as has also ethanol[76, 124], although

90

doubt has been cast that the latter's beneficial effect is really due to enzyme induction[36].

Anticonvulsants

Enzyme induction is of some consequence to epileptic patients, many of whom are treated with both phenobarbitone and phenytoin. The former increases metabolism of the latter[60] and lowers its steady-state plasma concentrations[23]. The effect of phenytoin, however, is to increase concentrations of phenobarbitone[75], probably as a result of inhibition of its breakdown. This is an interesting observation because phenytoin was thought to be an enzyme inducer (not the reverse) in man, largely because it accelerates hydroxylation of endogenous cortisol[128]. The latter effect may, however, be a consequence of excess cortisol production[129] and thus greater substrate availability rather than of an inducing action.

A further complication of anticonvulsant therapy is due to rapid breakdown (and inactivation) of vitamin D. Hahn and his colleagues[42] have demonstrated that vitamin D_3 and its active metabolite, 25-hydroxycholecalciferol, disappear abnormally rapidly from plasma following phenobarbitone treatment. This observation is consistent with the finding that plasma levels of the metabolite are abnormally low in a high proportion of treated epileptic patients[111]. Such deficiency is probably an important contributory cause of the overt osteomalacia which is sometimes found[28, 61] and of the decreased serum calcium concentrations[52] and reduced bone density[19] which appear to occur quite commonly in this situation. It has been suggested that induction may contribute to the folate deficiency which accompanies phenytoin administration[72], although there must also be other mechanisms involved.

Tolerance

Some degree of tolerance is common following chronic consumption of some non-barbiturate hypnotics and of ethanol. Many such agents induce their own metabolizing enzymes and this may be the origin of the tolerance which occurs. Glutethimide accelerates its own breakdown[102] and the metabolism of dipyrone to 4-aminoantipyrine[93], while meprobamate also accelerates its own breakdown[31]. The drug mixture of diphenhydramine and methaqualone (Mandrax) accelerates antipyrine metabolism after three weeks' administration to volunteers[112] and also in drug addicts[3], but whether it affects the breakdown of its components is not known. Nitrazepam appears not to induce enzymes at ordinary therapeutic dosage[112], nor does it influence anticoagulation by phenprocoumon[6] or warfarin[82]. Nitrazepam therefore appears to be the only safe hypnotic among those currently available to use if enzyme induction is to be avoided. Tolerance to opiate analgesics is not associated with enzyme induction in animals[93] and there is no reason to suspect that the enormous degree of tolerance which is shown by addicts has much to do with liver microsomal adaptation, although adaptive changes may well be found in the brain which could be critical.

Ethanol

The effects of ethanol administration on drug metabolism are complex. Acute doses large enough to keep blood concentrations in the region of 0.5–1.0 mg/ml prolong the half-lives of phenobarbitone and meprobamate[98], an action which is probably sufficient to account for the well known potentiation which occurs when such drugs are consumed together. A persistent high intake of ethanol also raises steady-state plasma warfarin concentrations with resultant increased anticoagulation *(Figure 7.5)*. On the other hand, chronic administration reduces neonatal hyperbilirubinaemia, an effect which has been ascribed to induction of glucuronidation, and it accelerates antipyrine[120], pentobarbitone and meprobamate[74] breakdown. Chronic administration has also been found to increase pentobarbitone hydroxylase activity twofold in liver biopsy specimens of three healthy volunteers[99] The effect on its own metabolism is somewhat irregular (see review by Hawkins and Kalant[48]). Although many alcoholics appear to metabolize the drug more rapidly than normal subjects, others do not show this effect and some show the opposite, perhaps because of severe liver damage. Among six healthy volunteers, Vesell, Page and Passananti[120] reported that three weeks' administration led to an increase in metabolism in three subjects but a decrease in the other three. A likely explanation of these findings lies in the fact that ethanol is metabolized by a number of different enzyme systems[48], by alcohol dehydrogenase and catalase as well as the microsomal mixed-function oxidases, which respond differently to the drug. There is therefore some doubt as to whether acquired tolerance to ethanol is the result of enzyme induction or not. As seems likely with barbiturates, adaptation may well occur in the central nervous system, too. Indeed, such adaptation has been demonstrated over a short period by Mirsky and his colleagues[73], who showed that eight subjects who were intoxicated within two hours of starting the drinking were sober hours later with blood alcohol concentrations higher than when they were drunk.

Environment

Environmental factors other than drugs may also cause enzyme induction. Kolmodin, Azarnoff and Sjöqvist[58] and Poland and his colleagues[85] have indicated that exposure to chlorinated insecticides such as dicophane and lindane accelerates antipyrine, phenylbutazone

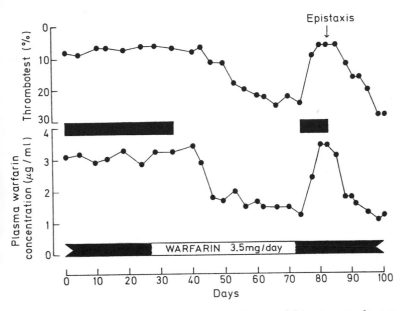

Figure 7.5. The effect of ethanol consumption (upper solid bars) on steady-state plasma warfarin concentrations and thrombotest activity in a patient receiving warfarin 3.5 mg/day. (From Breckenridge and Orme, 1971[8])

and cortisol breakdown, and recently a combination of town dwelling and cigarette smoking has been found to increase pentazocine requirements in anaesthetized subjects[56], a finding which is consistent with enzyme induction by hydrocarbons and benzpyrenes which certainly are powerful inducers in animals. Factory workers exposed to endrin excrete abnormally large amounts of 6β-hydroxycortisol[54] and glucaric acid[53], probably also indicating enzyme induction. Aldrin and dieldrin appear to lack this property. Cigarette smoking on its own accelerates nicotine metabolism, presumably by inducing the required enzyme[4], and it also stimulates benzpyrene-metabolizing enzymes in the human placenta[127]. Furthermore, a recent study by Pantuck,

Kuntzman and Conney[83] suggests that heavy smoking accelerates the disappearance of phenacetin from the body, again suggesting enzyme induction.

Extrahepatic tissues

Other tissues apart from the liver may also be susceptible to enzyme induction. Houck and Sharma[50] showed that human fibroblasts respond to a number of anti-inflammatory drugs by increasing collagenolytic and proteolytic activity, which could be of therapeutic importance. Of interest, too, is the curious observation[5] that methotrexate causes an increase in blood cell dihydrofolate reductase, the enzyme which it inhibits. The activity of this larger amount of enzyme remains inhibited, however, because of the stability of the drug–enzyme complex. It is perhaps worth speculating whether similar effects arise with other drugs (such as hydrazide monoamine oxidase inhibitors) which form particularly tight bonds with macromolecules.

Enzyme induction clearly plays an important part in drug therapy but it may also have a wider role in biology. Wilson[132] has shown that cultures of human myometrium respond to the presence of oestrogen by induction of malate dehydrogenase, a finding which lends support to the contention that many hormones exert their effects on the tissues of the body by induction (or, in some instances, repression) of vital enzyme systems. Induction and repression may also be important factors in the regulation of transmitter synthesis by negative feedback in the central and peripheral nervous systems and in some of the adaptive changes, such as increases in histamine-forming capacity, which occur in the inflammatory response.

Enzyme inhibition

Inhibition of drug metabolism by one drug may lead to the accumulation of other simultaneously administered drugs. The results of this process could give rise to even more serious clinical consequences than those seen with enzyme induction. At the present time, the number of drugs known to produce enzyme inhibition is very much smaller than that known to produce enzyme induction, but this situation may alter considerably. Many drugs are used in clinical medicine for their ability to inhibit enzymes; these include phenelzine and tranylcypromine (monoamine oxidase inhibitors), allopurinol (a xanthine oxidase inhibitor) and disulfiram (an aldehyde dehydrogenase inhibitor). Recent studies, however, suggest that these drugs inhibit many more enzymes than their so-called 'specificity' would suggest. Indeed, the statement that '... the specificity of an [enzyme] inhibitor is inversely proportional to its familiarity'[25] is truly appropriate.

The mechanisms by which drugs produce enzyme inhibition are poorly understood. In theory, inhibition could arise from any of the following.

(1) *Substrate competition:* two drugs, each of which is usually metabolized by the same enzyme, compete.

(2) *Competitive or non-competitive inhibition:* a substance which is not necessarily a substrate reduces the affinity or activity of the enzyme for its substrate.

(3) *Product inhibition:* the product of the enzyme reaction competes with the substrate.

(4) *Repression:* the amount of enzyme is reduced, either by decreased formation or by increased destruction.

The last-named process would probably take longer to develop and longer to decay than the others, although non-competitive enzyme inhibition by such drugs as monoamine oxidase inhibitors can also be long-lasting. In practice the mechanism can often be deduced only from animal experiments which may not apply to the clinical situation. Furthermore, the observation that one drug increases the half-life of an other completely metabolized drug does not necessarily mean that the drug is producing enzyme inhibition; an increase in the apparent volume of distribution without any change in clearance could also cause an increase in half-life (see Chapter 2). A further problem in studying enzyme inhibition is exemplified by SKF 525-A. This compound has been studied extensively in animals since it slows the metabolism of a wide variety of drugs including phenylbutazone, phenacetin and hexobarbitone when given as a single dose. Repeated administration, however, results in enzyme induction, a phenomenon which could result from positive feedback. Other examples of drugs which in animals appear to behave similarly are chlorcyclizine, phenylbutazone and glutethimide[13].

Drugs which have been reported to produce inhibition of metabolism of other drugs are listed in Table 7.2. Disulfiram, which inhibits ethanol metabolism at the acetaldehyde stage, prolongs antipyrine half-lives[123] and has been reported to raise steady-state plasma concentrations of warfarin[97] and phenytoin[77] and to increase the actions of these drugs clinically. The implication is that disulfiram inhibits microsomal enzyme activity. A study of two patients under treatment with phenytoin, however, revealed that the drug, while elevating plasma levels, did not reduce urinary excretion of hydroxyphenytoin, the principal metabolite[78]. The nature of the drug interaction is therefore unclear. Similar observations on the anticonvulsant drug, sulthiame, as an inhibitor of phenytoin metabolism[79] make it difficult to see why this drug also raises plasma phenytoin levels[45]. One possible explanation is that phenytoin is metabolized in more than one way and that disulfiram and sulthiame are inhibitors of subsidiary pathways. Calcium carbimide, which is used clinically as a substitute for disulfiram, does not appear to influence phenytoin concentrations.

TABLE 7.2. Substances Known to Cause Inhibition of Drug Metabolism in Man

Allopurinol	Nortriptyline
(Chloral hydrate)	Oral contraceptives
Chloramphenicol	Oxyphenbutazone
Dicoumarol	Para-aminosalicylate
Disulfiram	Perphenazine
Isoniazid	Phenylbutazone
Levodopa + methyldopa hydrazine	Phenyramidol
Methandrostenolone	Sulphaphenazole
Monoamine oxidase inhibitors	Sulthiame

Anticoagulant drugs of the coumarin type can enter into substrate competition with other drugs with resultant increase in their anticoagulant actions[57]. At the same time, anticoagulants can also potentiate other drugs. Thus dicoumarol prolongs the plasma half-life of phenytoin *(Figure 7.6)* and must be expected to precipitate toxic reactions in susceptible subjects. It also has a powerful potentiating action on tolbutamide[59].

Chemotherapeutic agents inhibit some drug-metabolizing pathways. In particular, chloramphenicol, a non-competitive inhibitor of microsomal enzymes in animals[29], inhibits both tolbutamide[18] and chlorpropamide[84] breakdown with resultant increased hypoglycaemia. Sulphaphenazole has similar actions in tolbutamide-treated diabetics[17, 104]. Phenytoin hydroxylation is inhibited in patients undergoing antituberculous chemotherapy[64], an effect which is probably caused by isoniazid accumulation[10]. Inactivation of isoniazid itself is reduced by PAS[44], a finding which may account in part for the beneficial effect of this drug in the treatment of tuberculosis.

Perhaps the most interesting observations on inhibition of drug metabolism are those of Vesell, Passananti and Greene[122] that half-lives of antipyrine and dicoumarol are prolonged by repeated administration of allopurinol or nortriptyline. Animal work indicated that the effect was caused by enzyme repression. The observations are not fully

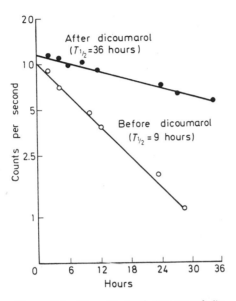

Figure 7.6. The effect of dicoumarol (in dosage sufficient to reduce prothrombin activity to 30 per cent of normal) on disposal of ^{14}C-phenytoin in one subject. (From Hansen, Kristensen, Skovsted and Christensen, 1966[46])

substantiated by subsequent work[80, 108] although with allopurinol some inhibitory effect is apparent. In spite of this the drug did not alter steady-state plasma levels in three patients on phenylbutazone and two on warfarin[108], which suggests that inhibition by allopurinol in many patients may be slight enough to be of little consequence.

Prolongation of half-lives and elevation of plasma levels have been reported with a number of other drugs. Methylphenidate, a structural analogue of SKF 525-A (mentioned above), has been reported to inhibit drug metabolism[37] but subsequent work has disproved this[63]. Phenothiazines and haloperidol[40], phenyramidol[109], oxyphenbutazone and methandrostenolone[126], oral contraceptive agents[81, 100] and some antiparkinson drugs[118], have also been found to inhibit drug oxidation but the significance of these observations remains to be established.

Monoamine oxidase (MAO) inhibitors

Drug interactions occur commonly with MAO inhibitors but their explanation is not always clear. They potentiate some sympathomimetics in man[34] and the hypertensive crises which follow administration of sympathomimetic amines, particularly those contained in cheese and other foods, are obviously related to inhibition of MAO. Thus inhibition of the enzyme in the intestinal wall and in the liver allows substances such as tyramine to escape their usual first-pass destruction and there is a resultant pressor effect. Strangely, there appears to be considerable variability in individual susceptibility to 'cheese headaches', some patients reporting that they have often eaten cheese without ill-effect. This may be explained by the finding[89] that in at least one variety of cheese the tyramine is localized to a region close to the rind *(Figure 7.7)*. Susceptibility to the adverse effects of cheese

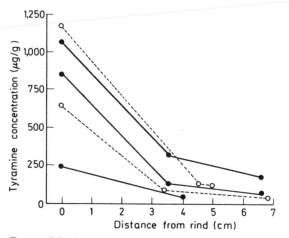

Figure 7.7. Tyramine content of Gruyère cheese in different positions in relation to the rind. (From Price and Smith, 1971[89])

consumption therefore depends on which part of the cheese is eaten. Some recent work suggests that susceptibility to 'cheese headaches' may be associated also with inability of the individual to metabolize tyramine by subsidiary chemical pathways[101].

It is often stated that MAO inhibitors inhibit microsomal enzymes in man as they do in animals[65, 90] but these statements do not appear to have been verified. Apparent toxicities of imipramine[68] and amylobarbitone[30] in the presence of tranylcypromine (a MAO inhibitor) have been reported in two individual patients. In one case, however, gross overdosage was involved and in the other trauma occurred which probably contributed to the apparent intoxication. Mebanazine (a MAO inhibitor of the hydrazide group) has been found to precipitate hypoglycaemic attacks in an insulin-treated diabetic patient[22], an action which is thought to have arisen from reduction of compensatory adrenergic responses[21].

The adverse reactions to pethidine which occur occasionally in patients taking MAO inhibitors are probably not due to inhibition of MAO. It also seems unlikely that they are due to inhibition of microsomal enzymes, unless qualitatively different metabolic pathways are involved, because the reactions (usually involving hypertension and hyperpyrexia) are so unlike those of an overdose. Morphine is commonly stated to be contraindicated in patients taking MAO inhibitors, although only one untoward reaction has been reported[110]. This whole subject urgently needs investigation.

Liver disease

It would seem likely that patients with liver damage should show impaired metabolism of drugs and consequent intolerance. Yet the evidence for this is somewhat conflicting. Essentially normal plasma half-lives of pentobarbitone[106], and of antipyrine, dicoumarol, salicylate and phenylbutazone[11], have been found in patients with cirrhosis. In a more recent study, Levi, Sherlock and Walker[66] revealed that many patients with liver disease who were not taking inducing agents had isoniazid and phenylbutazone half-lives which fell within the normal range. An association was found, however, between prolongation of the phenylbutazone half-life and the degree of impairment of liver function as indicated by the plasma albumin and aspartate transaminase levels. A similar impairment of amylobarbitone metabolism in association with hypoalbuminaemia has also been reported[71]. Cirrhotic patients metabolize chloramphenicol slowly[62] and erythropoietic depression occurring as a complication of chloramphenicol treatment has been found in 8 of 16 patients with liver disease but in none of 16 healthy patients[113]. In each case of toxicity, blood chloramphenicol levels were high, presumably because of impaired destruction by hepatic conjugating enzymes. Rifamycin[1] and tolbutamide[117] are also broken down more slowly in patients with liver disease and the latter drug produces a greater degree of hypoglycaemia. Confirmation that impairment of metabolism occurs only in severe liver disease comes from the work of Schoene and his colleagues[103] which has shown that liver biopsy specimens from such patients contain less cytochrome P-450 than normal and have less aminopyrine demethylase and pseudocholinesterase. Plasma of patients with severe liver disease also has less cholinesterase activity[91].

Patients poisoned with paracetamol may develop acute hepatic necrosis and in these individuals the rate of paracetamol metabolism is slowed. The paracetamol half-life in this situation provides a good prognostic guide[88]. Abnormally slow metabolism of barbiturates, phenytoin and antipyrine has also been observed in such patients[86].

Anaesthetists recognize that patients with liver disease require less thiopentone for anaesthesia than do healthy subjects[32, 107] but it seems likely that this arises not from slow thiopentone metabolism but from impaired binding to plasma albumin. In such patients albumin levels are low and the reduced number of binding sites may also be occupied by bilirubin which is present in abnormally high concentration. Impairment of lignocaine metabolism in severe cardiac failure from myocardial infarction has been ascribed to liver damage[87] although it seems probable that the impairment arises at least partially because of reduced liver blood flow.

Surprisingly, most patients with liver disease appear to respond normally to drugs such as barbiturates which cause enzyme induction[66]. Clearly, quite severe degrees of functional impairment must be present before the individual fails to respond to drug administration in a normal manner.

Renal disease

Certain pathways of drug metabolism are impaired in patients with uraemia. These include the acetylation of sulphafurazole[92], the reduction of cortisol[35] and the hydrolysis of esters by plasma pseudocholinesterase[91]. The mechanisms of these alterations are unclear but it appears that the diminished pseudocholinesterase activity of uraemic plasma is not due to competition by some unexcreted waste product. By contrast, the metabolism of phenytoin appears to be enhanced in uraemic patients[69], which is partly (though not completely) due to the reduction in protein binding of this drug which occurs with advancing renal failure (see Chapter 4).

References

1. Acocella, G., Baroni, G. C. and Muschio, R. (1962). 'Clinical evaluation of the therapeutic activity of rifamycin SV in the treatment of biliary tract infections.' *G. Mal. infett. parassit.* **14**, 552–555

2. Alexanderson, B., Evans, D. A. P. and Sjöqvist, F. (1969). 'Steady-state plasma levels of nortriptyline in twins: influence of genetic factors and drug therapy.' *Br. med. J.* **4**, 764–768

3. Ballinger, B., Browning, M., O'Malley, K. and Stevenson, I. H. (1972). 'Drug-metabolizing capacity in states of drug dependence and withdrawal.' *Br. J. Pharmac.* **45**, 638–643

4. Beckett, A. H. and Triggs, E. J. (1967). 'Enzyme induction in man caused by smoking.' *Nature, Lond.* **216**, 587

5. Bertino, J. R., Cashmore, A., Fink, M., Calabresi, P. and Lefkowitz, E. (1965). 'The "induction" of leukocyte and erythrocyte dihydrofolate reductase by methotrexate. II. Clinical and pharmacologic studies.' *Clin. Pharmac. Ther.* **6**, 763–770

6. Bieger, R., Jonge, H. de and Loeliger, E. A. (1972). 'Influence of nitrazepam on oral anticoagulation with phenprocoumon.' *Clin. Pharmac. Ther.* **13**, 361–365

7. Breckenridge, A. (1972). Personal communication

8. Breckenridge, A. and Orme, M. (1971). 'Clinical implications of enzyme induction.' *Ann. N.Y. Acad. Sci.* **179**, 421–431

9. Breckenridge, A., Orme, M.L'E., Thorgeirsson, S., Davies, D. S. and Brooks, R. V. (1971). 'Drug interactions with warfarin: studies with dichloralphenazone, chloral hydrate and phenazone (antipyrine).' *Clin. Sci.* **40**, 351–364

10. Brennan, R. W., Dehejia, H., Kutt, H. and McDowell, F. (1968). 'Diphenylhydantoin intoxication attendant to slow inactivation of isoniazid.' *Neurology, Minneap.* **18**, 283

11. Brodie, B. B., Burns, J. J. and Weiner, M. (1959). 'Metabolism of drugs in subjects with Laennec's cirrhosis.' *Medna exp.* **1**, 290–292

12. Brooks, S. M., Werk, E. E., Ackerman, S. J., Sullivan, I. and Thrasher, K. (1972). 'Adverse effects of phenobarbital on corticosteroid metabolism in patients with bronchial asthma.' *New Engl. J. Med.* **286**, 1125–1128

13. Burns, J. J. and Conney, A. H. (1965). 'Enzyme stimulation and inhibition in the metabolism of drugs.' *Proc. R. Soc. Med.* **58**, 955–960

14. Burstein, S. and Klaiber, E. L. (1965). 'Phenobarbital-induced increase in 6-beta-hydroxycortisol excretion: clue to its significance in human urine.' *J. clin. Endocr. Metab.* **25**, 293–296

15. Busfield, D., Child, K. J., Atkinson, R. M. and Tomich, E. G. (1963). 'An effect of phenobarbitone on blood-levels of griseofulvin in man.' *Lancet* **2**, 1042–1043

16. Catalano, P. M. and Cullen, S. I. (1966). 'Warfarin antagonism by griseofulvin.' *Clin. Res.* **14**, 266

17. Christensen, L. K., Hansen, J. M. and Kristensen, M. (1963). 'Sulphaphenazole-induced hypoglycaemic attacks in tolbutamide-treated diabetics.' *Lancet* **2**, 1298–1301

18. Christensen, L. K. and Skovsted, L. (1969). 'Inhibition of drug metabolism by chloramphenicol.' *Lancet* **2**, 1397–1399

19. Christiansen, C., Kristensen, M. and Rødbro, P. (1972). 'Latent osteomalacia in epileptic patients on anticonvulsants.' *Br. med. J.* **3**, 738–739

20. Conney, A. H. (1967). 'Pharmacological implications of microsomal enzyme induction.' *Pharmac. Rev.* **19**, 317–366

21. Cooper, A. J. and Ashcroft, G. (1966). 'Potentiation of insulin hypoglycaemia by M.A.O.I. antidepressant drugs.' *Lancet* **1**, 407–409

22. Cooper, A. J. and Keddie, K. M. G. (1964). 'Hypotensive collapse and hypoglycaemia after mebanazine – a monoamine-oxidase inhibitor.' *Lancet* **1**, 1133–1135

23. Cucinell, S. A., Conney, A. H., Sansur, M. and Burns, J. J. (1965). 'Drug interactions in man. 1. Lowering effect of phenobarbital on plasma levels of bishydroxycoumarin (Dicumarol) and diphenylhydantoin (Dilantin).' *Clin. Pharmac. Ther.* **6**, 420–429

24. Cucinell, S. A., Odessky, L., Weiss, M. and Dayton, P. G. (1966). 'The effect of chloral hydrate on bishydroxycoumarin metabolism.' *J. Am. med. Ass.* **197**, 366–368

25. Davenport, H. W. (1962). 'Carbonic anhydrase inhibition and physiological function.' In *Enzymes and Drug Action*, p. 16. Ciba Foundation Symposium. Ed. by J. L. Mongar and A. V. S. de Reuck. Edinburgh and London: Churchill Livingstone

26. Davies, J. E., Edmundson, W. F., Carter, C. H. and Barquet, A. (1969). 'Effect of anticonvulsant drugs on dicophane (D.D.T.) residues in man.' *Lancet* **2**, 7–9

27. Dayton, P. G., Tarcan, Y., Chenkin, T. and Weiner, M. (1961). 'The influence of barbiturates on coumarin plasma levels and prothrombin response.' *J. clin. Invest.* **40**, 1797–1802

28. Dent, C. E., Richens, A., Rowe, D. J. F. and Stamp, T. C. B. (1970). 'Osteomalacia with long-term anticonvulsant therapy in epilepsy.' *Br. med. J.* **4**, 69–72

29. Dixon, R. L. and Fouts, J. R. (1962). 'Inhibition of microsomal drug metabolic pathways by chloramphenicol.' *Biochem. Pharmac.* **11**, 715–720

30. Domino, E. F., Sullivan, T. S. and Luby, E. D. (1962). 'Barbiturate intoxication in a patient treated with a MAO inhibitor.' *Am. J. Psychiat.* **118**, 941–943

31. Douglas, J. F., Ludwig, B. J. and Smith, N. (1963). 'Studies on the metabolism of meprobamate.' *Proc. Soc. exp. Biol. Med.* **112**, 436–438

32. Dundee, J. W. (1952). 'Thiopentone narcosis in the presence of hepatic dysfunction.' *Br. J. Anaesth.* **24**, 81–100

33. Ebert, A. G., Yim, G. K. W. and Miya, T. C. (1964). 'Distribution and metabolism of barbital-^{14}C in tolerant and nontolerant rats.' *Biochem. Pharmac.* **13**, 1267–1274

34. Elis, J., Laurence, D. R., Mattie, H. and Prichard, B. N. C.

(1967). 'Modification by monoamine oxidase inhibitors of the effect of some sympathomimetics on blood pressure.' *Br. med. J.* **2**, 75–78

35. Englert, E., Brown, H., Willardson, D. G., Wallach, S. and Simons, E. L. (1958). 'Metabolism of free and conjugated 17-hydroxycorticosteroids in subjects with uremia.' *J. clin. Endocr. Metab.* **18**, 36–48

36. Garbagnati, E. and Manitto, P. (1972). 'Possible interaction of ethanol with unconjugated bilirubin in jaundiced subjects.' *Lancet* **1**, 693

37. Garrettson, L. K., Perel, J. M. and Dayton, P. G. (1969). 'Methylphenidate interaction with both anticonvulsants and ethyl biscoumacetate: a new action of methylphenidate.' *J. Am. med. Ass.* **207**, 2053–2056

38. Gerald, M. C. and Feller, D. R. (1970). 'Stimulation of barbiturate metabolism by spironolactone in mice.' *Archs int. Pharmacodyn. Thér.* **187**, 120–124

39. Goss, J. E. and Dickhaus, D. W. (1965). 'Increased bishydroxy-coumarin requirements in patients receiving phenobarbital.' *New Engl. J. Med.* **273**, 1094–1095

40. Gram, L. F. and Overø, K. F. (1972). 'Drug interaction: inhibitory effect of neuroleptics on metabolism of tricyclic antidepressants in man.' *Br. med. J.* **1**, 463–465

41. Granick, S. (1966). 'The induction *in vitro* of the synthesis of δ-amino-levulinic acid synthetase in chemical porphyria: a response to certain drugs, sex hormones and foreign chemicals.' *J. biol. Chem.* **241**, 1359–1375

42. Hahn, T. J., Birge, S. J., Scharp, C. R. and Avioli, L. V. (1972). 'Phenobarbital-induced alterations in vitamin D metabolism.' *J. clin. Invest.* **51**, 741–748

43. Hammer, W., Ideström, C.-M. and Sjöqvist, F. (1967). 'Chemical control of antidepressant drug therapy.' In *Anti-Depressant Drugs*, Excerpta Medica Int. Congr. Series **122**, pp. 301–310. Amsterdam: Excerpta Medica

44. Hanngren, Å., Borgå, O. and Sjöqvist, F. (1970). 'Inactivation of isoniazid (INH) in Swedish tuberculous patients before and during treatment with para-aminosalicylic acid (PAS).' *Scand. J. resp. Dis.* **51**, 61–69

45. Hansen, J. M., Kristensen, M. and Skovsted, L. (1968). 'Sulthiame (Ospolot) as inhibitor of diphenylhydantoin metabolism.' *Epilepsia* **9**, 17–22

46. Hansen, J. M., Kristensen, M. D., Skovsted, L. and Christensen, L. K. (1966). 'Dicoumarol-induced diphenylhydantoin intoxication.' *Lancet* **2**, 265–266

47. Hansen, J. M., Siersbaek-Nielsen, K. and Skovsted, L. (1971). 'Carbamazepine-induced acceleration of diphenylhydantoin and warfarin metabolism in man.' *Clin. Pharmac. Ther.* **12**, 539–543

48. Hawkins, R. D. and Kalant, H. (1972). 'The metabolism of ethanol and its metabolic effects.' *Pharmac. Rev.* **24**, 67–157

49. Hoogland, D. R., Miya, T. S. and Bousquet, W. F. (1966). 'Metabolism and tolerance studies with chlordiazepoxide-2-^{14}C in the rat.' *Toxic. appl. Pharmac.* **9**, 116–123

50. Houck, J. C. and Sharma, V. K. (1968). 'Induction of collagenolytic and proteolytic activities in rat and human fibroblasts by anti-inflammatory drugs.' *Science, N.Y.* **161**, 1361–1362

51. Hunter, J., Maxwell, J. D., Carrella, M., Stewart, D. A. and Williams, R. (1971). 'Urinary D-glucaric acid excretion as a test for hepatic enzyme induction in man.' *Lancet* **1**, 572–575

52. Hunter, J., Maxwell, J. D., Stewart, D. A., Parsons, V. and Williams, R. (1971). 'Altered calcium metabolism in epileptic children on anticonvulsants.' *Br. med. J.* **4**, 202–204

53. Hunter, J., Maxwell, J. D., Stewart, D. A., Williams, R., Robinson, J. and Richardson, A. (1972). 'Increased hepatic microsomal enzyme activity from occupational exposure to certain organochlorine pesticides.' *Nature, Lond.* **237**, 399–401

54. Jager, K. W. (1970). *Aldrin, Dieldrin, Endrin and Telodrin: an epidemiological and toxicological study of long term occupational exposure.* Amsterdam and London: Elsevier

55. Jelliffe, R. W. and Blankenhorn, D. H. (1966). 'Effects of phenobarbital on digitoxin metabolism.' *Clin. Res.* **14**, 160

56. Keeri-Szanto, M. and Pomeroy, J. R. (1971). 'Atmospheric pollution and pentazocine metabolism.' *Lancet* **1**, 947–949

57. Koch-Weser, J. and Sellers, E. M. (1971). 'Drug interactions with coumarin anticoagulants.' *New Engl. J. Med.* **285**, 487–498; 547–558

58. Kolmodin, B., Azarnoff, D. L. and Sjöqvist, F. (1969). 'Effect of environmental factors on drug metabolism: decreased plasma half-life of antipyrine in workers exposed to chlorinated insecticides.' *Clin. Pharmac. Ther.* **10**, 638–642

59. Kristensen, M. D. and Hansen, J. M. (1967). 'Potentiation of the tolbutamide effect by dicoumarol.' *Diabetes* **16**, 211–214

60. Kristensen, M. D., Hansen, J. M. and Skovsted, L. (1969). 'The influence of phenobarbital on the half-life of diphenylhydantoin in man.' *Acta med. scand.* **185**, 347–350

61. Kruse, R. (1968). 'Osteopathien bei antiepileptischer Langzeittherapie.' *Mschr. Kinderheilk.* **116**, 378–380

62. Kunin, C. M., Glazko, A. J. and Finland, M. (1959). 'Persistence of antibiotics in blood of patients with acute renal failure. II. Chloramphenicol and its metabolic products in the blood of patients with severe renal disease or hepatic cirrhosis.' *J. clin. Invest.* **38**, 1498–1508

63. Kupferberg, H. J., Jeffery, W. and Hunninghake, D. B. (1972). 'Effect of methylphenidate on plasma anticonvulsant levels.' *Clin. Pharmac. Ther.* **13**, 201–204

64. Kutt, H., Winters, W. and McDowell, F. H. (1966). 'Depression of para-hydroxylation of diphenylhydantoin by antituberculous chemotherapy.' *Neurology, Minneap.* **16**, 594–602

65. Laroche, M-J. and Brodie, B. B. (1960). 'Lack of relationship between inhibition of monoamine oxidase and potentiation of hexobarbital hypnosis.' *J. Pharmac. exp. Ther.* **130**, 134–137

66. Levi, A. J., Sherlock, S. and Walker, D. (1968). 'Phenylbutazone and isoniazid metabolism in patients with liver disease in relation to previous drug therapy.' *Lancet* **1**, 1275–1279

67. Long, R. F. (1969). 'Induction of drug-metabolizing enzymes and cytochrome P-450.' *Biochem. J.* **115**, 26P

68. Luby, E. D. and Domino, E. F. (1961). 'Toxicity from large doses of imipramine and an MAO inhibitor in suicidal intent.' *J. Am. med. Ass.* **177**, 68–69

69. Lund, L., Lunde, P. K., Rane, A., Borgå, O. and Sjöqvist, F. (1971). 'Plasma protein binding, plasma concentrations, and effects of diphenylhydantoin in man.' *Ann. N.Y. Acad. Sci.* **179**, 723–728

70. Maurer, H. M., Wolff, J. A., Finster, M., Poppers, P. J., Pantuck, E., Kuntzman, R. and Conney, A. H. (1968). 'Reduction in concentration of total serum-bilirubin in offspring of women treated with phenobarbitone during pregnancy.' *Lancet* **2**, 122–124

71. Mawer, G. E., Miller, N. E. and Turnberg, L. A. (1972). 'Metabolism of amylobarbitone in patients with chronic liver disease.' *Br. J. Pharmac.* **44**, 549–560

72. Maxwell, J. D., Hunter, J., Stewart, D. A., Ardeman, S. and Williams, R. (1972). 'Folate deficiency after anticonvulsant drugs: an effect of hepatic enzyme induction.' *Br. med. J.* **1**, 297–299

73. Mirsky, I. A., Piker, P., Rosenbaum, M. and Lederer, H. (1941). ' "Adaptation" of the central nervous system to varying concentrations of alcohol in the blood.' *Q. Jl Stud. Alcohol* **2**, 35–45

74. Misra, P. S., Lefèvre, A., Ishii, H., Rubin, E. and Lieber, C. S. (1971). 'Increase of ethanol, meprobamate and pentobarbital metabolism after chronic ethanol administration in man and in rats.' *Am. J. Med.* **51**, 346–351

75. Morselli, P. L., Rizzo, M. and Garattini, S. (1971). 'Interaction between phenobarbital and diphenylhydantoin in animals and in epileptic patients.' *Ann. N.Y. Acad. Sci.* **179**, 88–107

76. Okolicsanyi, L., Cartei, G. and Naccarato, R. (1972). 'Effects of ethanol on Gilbert's hyperbilirubinaemia.' *Lancet* **1**, 450

77. Olesen, O. V. (1966). 'Disulfiramum (Antabuse) as inhibitor of phenytoin metabolism.' *Acta Pharmac. Tox.* **24**, 317–322

78. Olesen, O. V. (1967). 'The influence of disulfiram and calcium carbimide on the serum diphenylhydantoin.' *Archs Neurol. Chicago,* **16**, 642–644

79. Olesen, O. V. and Jensen, O. N. (1969). 'Drug-interaction between sulthiame (Ospolot R) and phenytoin in the treatment of epilepsy.' *Dan. med. Bull.* **16**, 154—158

80. O'Malley, K., Sawyer, P. R., Stevenson, I. H. and Turnbull, M. J. (1972). 'Effects of tricyclic antidepressants on drug metabolism.' *Br. J. Pharmac.* **44**, 372—373P

81. O'Malley, K., Stevenson, I. H. and Crooks, J. (1972). 'Impairment of human drug metabolism by oral contraceptive steroids.' *Clin. Pharmac. Ther.* **13**, 552—557

82. Orme, M., Breckenridge, A. and Brooks, R. V. (1972). 'Interactions of benzodiazepines with warfarin.' *Br. med. J.* **3**, 611—614

83. Pantuck, E. J., Kuntzman, R. and Conney, A. H. (1972). 'Decreased concentration of phenacetin in plasma of cigarette smokers.' *Science, N.Y.* **175**, 1248—1250

84. Petitpierre, B. and Fabre, J. (1970). 'Chlorpropamide and chloramphenicol.' *Lancet* **1**, 789

85. Poland, A., Smith, D., Kuntzman, R., Jacobson, M. and Conney, A. H. (1970).. 'Effect of intensive occupational exposure to DDT on phenylbutazone and cortisol metabolism in human subjects.' *Clin. Pharmac. Ther.* **11**, 724—732

86. Prescott, L. F. (1972). 'The modifying effects of physiological variables and disease upon pharmacokinetics and/or drug response. Liver disease.' *Proc. 5th Int. Congr. Pharmac*, p. 73. Basle: Karger

87. Prescott, L. F. and Nimmo, J. (1971). 'Plasma lidocaine concentrations during and after prolonged infusions in patients with myocardial infarction.' In *Lidocaine in the Treatment of Ventricular Arrhythmias*, pp. 168—177. Ed. by D. B. Scott and D. G. Julian. Edinburgh and London: Churchill Livingstone

88. Prescott, L. F., Wright, N., Roscoe, P. and Brown, S. S. (1971). 'Plasma-paracetamol half-life and hepatic necrosis in patients with paracetamol overdosage.' *Lancet* **1**, 519—522

89. Price, K. and Smith, S. E. (1971). 'Cheese reaction and tyramine.' *Lancet* **1**, 130—131

90. Reber, K. and Studer, A. (1965). 'Beeinflussung der Wirkung einiger indirekter Antikoagulantien durch Monoaminoxydase-Hemmer.' *Thromb. Diath. haemorrh.* **14**, 83—87

91. Reidenberg, M. M., James, M. and Dring, L. G. (1972). 'The rate of procaine hydrolysis in serum of normal subjects and diseased patients.' *Clin. Pharmac. Ther.* **13**, 279—284

92. Reidenberg, M. M., Kostenbauder, H. and Adams, W. (1969). 'Rate of drug metabolism in obese volunteers before and during starvation and in azotemic patients.' *Metabolism* **18**, 209—213

93. Remmer, H. (1962). 'Drug tolerance.' In *Enzymes and Drug Action*, p. 276. Ciba Foundation Symposium. Ed. by J. L. Mongar and A. V. S. de Reuck. Edinburgh and London: Churchill Livingstone

94. Robinson, D. S. and Macdonald, M. G. (1966). 'The effect of phenobarbital administration on the control of coagulation achieved during warfarin therapy in man.' *J. Pharmac. exp. Ther.* **153**, 250−253

95. Robinson, D. S. and Sylvester, D. (1970). 'Interaction of commonly prescribed drugs and warfarin.' *Ann. intern. Med.* **72**, 853−856

96. Rosalki, S. B., Tarlow, D. and Rau, D. (1971). 'Plasma gamma-glutamyl transpeptidase elevation in patients receiving enzyme-inducing drugs.' *Lancet* **2**, 376−377

97. Rothstein, E. (1968). 'Warfarin effect enhanced by disulfiram.' *J. Am. med. Ass.* **206**, 1574−1575

98. Rubin, E., Gang, H., Misra, P. and Lieber, C. S. (1970). 'Inhibition of drug metabolism by acute intoxication: a hepatic microsomal mechanism.' *Am. J. Med.* **49**, 801−806

99. Rubin, E. and Lieber, C. S. (1968). 'Hepatic microsomal enzymes in man and rat − induction and inhibition by ethanol.' *Science, N.Y.* **162**, 690−691

100. Rudofsky, S. and Crawford, J. S. (1966). 'Some alterations in the pattern of drug metabolism associated with pregnancy, oral contraceptives and the newly-born.' *Pharmacologist* **8**, 181

101. Sandler, M. (1972). Personal communication

102. Schmid, K., Cornu, F., Imhof, P. and Keberle, H. (1964). 'Die biochemische Deutung der Gewohnung an Schlafmittel.' *Schweiz. med. Wschr.* **94**, 235−240

103. Schoene, B., Fleischmann, R. A., Remmer, H. and Oldershausen, H. F.v. (1972). 'Determination of drug metabolizing enzymes in needle biopsies of human liver.' *Eur. J. clin. Pharmac.* **4**, 65−73

104. Schulz, E. and Schmidt, F. H. (1970). 'Abbauhemmung von Tolbutamid durch Sulfaphenazol beim Menschen.' *Pharmacologia Clin.* **2**, 150−154

105. Sellers, E. M. and Koch-Weser, J. (1970). 'Potentiation of warfarin-induced hypoprothrombinaemia by chloral hydrate.' *New Engl. J. Med.* **283**, 827−831

106. Sessions, J. T., Minkel, H. P., Bullard, J. C. and Ingelfinger, F. J. (1954). 'The effect of barbiturates in patients with liver disease.' *J. clin. Invest.* **33**, 1116−1127

107. Shideman, F. E., Kelly, A. R., Lee, L. E., Lowell, V. F. and Adams, B. J. (1949). 'The role of the liver in the detoxication of thiopental (Pentothal) in man.' *Anesthesiology* **10**, 421−427

108. Smith, S. E. and Rawlins, M. D. (1973). 'Influence of allopurinol on drug metabolism in man.' *Br. J. Pharmac.* (in press)

109. Solomon, H. M. and Schrogie, J. J. (1967). 'The effect of phenyramidol on the metabolism of bishydroxycoumarin.' *Clin. Pharmac. Ther.* **8**, 554−556

110. Spencer, G. T. and Smith, S. E. (1963). 'Dangers of monoamine oxidase inhibitors.' *Br. med. J.* **1**, 750

111.   Stamp, T. C. B., Round, J. M., Rowe, D. J. F. and Haddad, J. G. (1972). 'Plasma levels and therapeutic effect of 25-hydroxy-cholecalciferol in epileptic patients taking anticonvulsant drugs.' *Br. med. J.* **4**, 9–12

112.   Stevenson, I. H. and O'Malley, K. (1972). 'Changes in human drug metabolising capacity following exposure to hypnotics.' *Proc. 5th Int. Congr. Pharmac.* p. 222. Basle: Karger

113.   Suhrland, L. G. and Weisberger, A. S. (1963). 'Chloramphenicol toxicity in liver and renal disease.' *Archs intern. Med.* **112**, 747–754

114.   Taylor, S. A., Rawlins, M. D. and Smith, S. E. (1972). 'Spirono-lactone – a weak enzyme inducer in man.' *J. Pharm. Pharmac.* **24**, 578–579

115.   Thompson, R. P. H., Stathers, G. M., Pilcher, C. W. T., McLean, A. E. M., Robinson, J. and Williams, R. (1969). 'Treatment of unconjugated jaundice with dicophane.' *Lancet* **2**, 4–6

116.   Trolle, D. (1968). 'Decrease of total serum-bilirubin concentration in newborn infants after phenobarbitone treatment.' *Lancet* **2**, 705–708

117.   Ueda, H., Sakurai, T., Ota, M., Nakajima, A., Kamii, K. and Maezawa, H. (1963). 'Disappearance rate of tolbutamide in normal subjects and in diabetes mellitus, liver cirrhosis and renal disease.' *Diabetes* **12**, 414–419

118.   Vesell, E. S., Ng, L., Passananti, G. T. and Chase, T. N. (1971). 'Inhibition of drug metabolism by levodopa in combination with a dopa-decarboxylase inhibitor.' *Lancet* **2**, 370

119.   Vesell, E. S. and Page, J. G. (1969). 'Genetic control of the phenobarbital-induced shortening of plasma antipyrine half-lives in man.' *J. clin. Invest.* **48**, 2202–2209

120.   Vesell, E. S., Page, J. G. and Passananti, G. T. (1971). 'Genetic and environmental factors affecting ethanol metabolism in man.' *Clin. Pharmac. Ther.* **12**, 192–201

121.   Vesell, E. S. and Passananti, G. T. (1972). 'Differential effects of chronic halofenate administration on drug metabolism in man.' *Fedn Proc.* **31**, 538

122.   Vesell, E. S., Passananti, G. T. and Greene, F. E. (1970). 'Impairment of drug metabolism in man by allopurinol and nortriptyline.' *New Engl. J. Med.* **283**, 1484–1488

123.   Vesell, E. S., Passananti, G. T. and Lee, C. H. (1971). 'Impairment of drug metabolism by disulfiram in man.' *Clin. Pharmac. Ther.* **12**, 785–792

124.   Waltman, R., Bonura, F., Nigrin, G. and Pipat, C. (1969). 'Ethanol in prevention of hyperbilirubinaemia in the newborn. A controlled trial.' *Lancet* **2**, 1265–1267

125.   Watson, M., Gabica, J. and Benson, W. W. (1972). 'Serum organochlorine pesticides in mentally retarded patients on differing drug regimens.' *Clin. Pharmac. Ther.* **13**, 186–192

126. Weiner, M., Siddiqui, A. A., Bostanci, N. and Dayton, P. G. (1965). 'Drug interactions: the effect of combined administration on the half-life of coumarin and pyrazolone drugs in man.' *Fedn Proc.* **24**, 153

127. Welch, R. M., Harrison, Y. E., Conney, A. H., Poppers, P. J. and Finster, M. (1968). 'Cigarette smoking: stimulatory effect on metabolism of 3,4-benzpyrene by enzymes in human placenta.' *Science, N.Y.* **160**, 541—542

128. Werk, E. E., MacGee, J. and Sholiton, L. J. (1964). 'Effect of diphenylhydantoin on cortisol metabolism in man.' *J. clin. Invest.* **43**, 1824—1835

129. Werk, E. E., Thrasher, K., Sholiton, L. J., Olinger, C. and Choi, Y. (1971). 'Cortisol production in epileptic patients treated with diphenylhydantoin.' *Clin. Pharmac. Ther.* **12**, 698—703

130. Whelton, M. J., Krustev, L. P. and Billing, B. H. (1968). 'Reduction in serum bilirubin by phenobarbital in adult unconjugated hyperbilirubinaemia. Is enzyme induction responsible?' *Am. J. med.* **45**, 160—164

131. Whittaker, J. A. and Evans, D. A. P. (1970). 'Genetic control of phenylbutazone metabolism in man.' *Br. med. J.* **4**, 323—328

132. Wilson, E. (1967). 'Induction of malate dehydrogenase by oestradiol-17β in the human myometrium.' *Nature, Lond.* **215**, 758—759

CHAPTER 8

Drug Excretion

Many drugs are eliminated, at least in part, by excretion in the urine and bile. Other routes of excretion such as saliva, sweat, milk, lacrimal and vaginal secretions are of only minor importance.

Renal excretion

The elimination of drugs by the kidney is dependent upon the net consequences of glomerular filtration, tubular secretion and tubular reabsorption.

Glomerular filtration is a passive process relying on the hydrostatic pressure gradient between the glomerular capillaries and the glomerular space. The only restriction is one of molecular size. Compounds of more than 60,000–70,000 molecular weight are unable to cross into the glomerular space, with the result that the glomerular fluid is essentially free of plasma proteins. Although most drugs are thus capable of crossing the glomerular membrane on the basis of size, drug molecules bound to protein in the plasma are excluded. Moreover, in contradistinction to the process of active tubular secretion (see below), the filtration process leaves the concentration of unbound drug in plasma water unaltered so that the equilibrium between bound and unbound drug is undisturbed. Protein binding therefore offers an important restriction to the glomerular filtration of drugs. Increases in the unbound fraction of drug, either from a reduction in plasma albumin or from displacement by other drugs, may result in increased renal elimination.

In the proximal tubule, both organic acids and bases are actively transported into the tubular fluid by the tubular cells. Separate 'pumps' are present for acids and bases. Although only the unbound drug in the plasma of the peritubular capillaries is available for secretion, the process disturbs the equilibrium between bound and unbound drug, result-

110

ing in dissociation of drug molecules from their carrier proteins in the plasma. As a result, both fractions appear in the urine. Although drugs that are actively secreted are also filtered at the glomerulus, secretion is clearly the more important process and it is customary to say that these drugs are 'excreted by active secretion'.

The anionic pump which secretes organic acids normally adds endogenous compounds such as uric acid to the tubular fluid. Drugs secreted by this mechanism are listed in Table 8.1. The transport mechanism is

TABLE 8.1. Drugs Undergoing Active Tubular Secretion

Acidic drugs	Basic drugs
Acetazolamide	Amiloride
Ampicillin	Dihydrocodeine
Benzylpenicillin	Hexamethonium
Cephaloridine	Mecamylamine
Cloxacillin	Morphine
Ethacrynic acid	Neostigmine
Frusemide	Pempidine
Indomethacin	Procaine
Mersalyl	Quinine
Phenylbutazone	Tolazoline
Probenecid	Triamterene
Salicylate	
Thiazide diuretics	

also responsible for the active secretion of some drug metabolites, particularly conjugates of glycine (e.g. salicylurate[34]), glucuronic acid (e.g. chloramphenicol glucuronide[21]) and sulphuric acid (e.g. morphine ethereal sulphate[41]). Since the acidic drugs in Table 8.1 share a common secretory mechanism in the proximal tubule, competition between various anions may produce a considerable decrease in renal clearance. Thus probenecid can be used to reduce the elimination rate of penicillins by competing for active tubular secretion. Much less desirable is the potentiation of acetohexamide hypoglycaemia following the administration of phenylbutazone[12]. Although the mechanism is unproven, it is probably due to the reduction in the tubular secretion of the former drug by the latter. Low doses of salicylate, probenecid and phenylbutazone block the tubular secretion of uric acid[43] and may precipitate gout; higher doses are needed to prevent the tubular re-absorption of uric acid in order to produce uricosuria. A similar mechanism is responsible for the hyperuricaemia and gout which may accompany the administration of frusemide, ethacrynic acid and thiazide diuretics. An acute attack of gout may also be produced during the initial stages of treatment with the xanthine oxidase inhibitor, allopurinol. The mechanism may be due to the fact that allopurinol undergoes metabolism to alloxanthine (oxypurinol) which competes with uric acid for tubular secretion[42]. When therapy has become established and uric acid production has been reduced by the action of allopurinol, this process becomes unimportant.

The separate cationic 'pump' responsible for the tubular secretion of organic bases has been the subject of comparatively little investigation. Drugs undergoing active transport across the tubular epithelium by this 'pump' are given in Table 8.1. Whether competition for tubular secretion between various bases is important in the renal excretion of drugs in man is uncertain, but animal experiments indicate that such a process might occur[40].

Diffusion of drugs occurs across the tubular cells of both the proximal and the distal tubules. Since the process is purely one of diffusion, drug molecules move from regions of higher concentration to regions of lower concentration. Although the mechanism is therefore potentially bidirectional the reabsorption of water and electrolytes creates a concentration gradient favouring the passage of drugs from the tubular fluid into the blood and net reabsorption results. An increase in urine flow reduces this concentration gradient and the time taken for such equilibration to occur and may increase the renal excretion of some drugs, particularly weak electrolytes. This fact is utilized in the treatment of barbiturate poisoning since there is a linear relationship between the renal clearances of butobarbitone, amylobarbitone, cyclobarbitone and phenobarbitone and urine flow[26] *(Figure 8.1)*.

The passive reabsorption of drugs across the epithelium of renal tubules involves passage through cell membranes and is therefore limited to lipid-soluble drugs and the non-ionized fraction of weak acids and bases. The same physicochemical principles involved in drug absorption (see Chapter 3) and drug distribution (see Chapter 4) therefore apply. Thus, for weak acids, increasing the pH of the tubular fluid increases the degree of ionization and so reduces drug reabsorption; for weak bases, increasing pH reduces the degree of ionization and favours reabsorption. In general, an acidic drug will show the phenomenon of pH-dependent excretion if the pK_a is within the range 3.0–7.5 and for a basic drug if the pK_a is between 7.5 and 10.5[27].

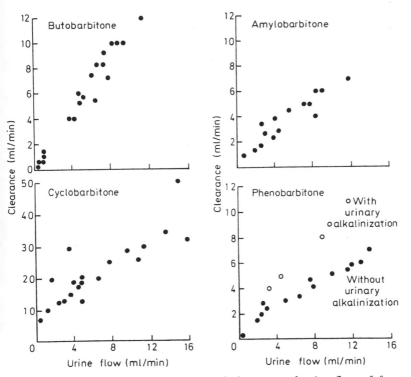

Figure 8.1. The relationship between renal clearance and urine flow of four barbiturates in man. In each case clearance increases linearly with increased urine flow. (From Linton, Luke and Briggs, 1967[26])

Thus, the renal excretion of weak acids (pK_a 3.0–7.5) is increased in an alkaline urine and the excretion of weak bases (pK_a 7.5–10.5) is increased in an acid urine. This is illustrated by the effect of changes in urine pH on the renal clearance of salicylate, a weak acid ($pK_a = 3.0$), as shown in *Figure 8.2*.

From a practical point of view, the importance of this process lies in the fact that changes in urinary pH may profoundly alter the elimination half-life ($T_{1/2}$) of those drugs undergoing appreciable renal excretion and which are weak electrolytes with pK_a values in the appropriate range. Examination of the details in Appendix C indicates those drugs for which this phenomenon is important. Sulphafurazole ($pK_a = 4.9$), which is largely excreted unchanged in the urine, has a $T_{1/2}$ of 9.5 hours at a urinary pH of 5 but a $T_{1/2}$ of 4.7 hours when the urinary pH is

113

8[10]. In contrast, although imipramine ($pK_a = 9.5$) can be shown to undergo pH-dependent excretion[5], the contribution of renal elimination of the drug is so small (less than 1 per cent) that urinary acidification does not produce an important change in $T_{1/2}$. In the treatment of

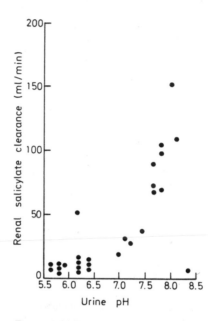

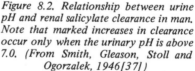

Figure 8.2. Relationship between urine pH and renal salicylate clearance in man. Note that marked increases in clearance occur only when the urinary pH is above 7.0. (From Smith, Gleason, Stoll and Ogorzalek, 1946[37])

poisoning, manipulation of urinary pH (combined with forced diuresis) increases the elimination rates of those drugs whose pK_a values lie in the appropriate range. Thus a forced alkaline diuresis increases the rate of elimination of salicylate[24], causing an approximately fourfold increase in clearance for each rise of 1 unit in urinary pH[28]. Forced alkaline diuresis is also of value in the management of patients with phenobarbitone intoxication ($pK_a = 7.2$) but altering urinary pH does not influence the elimination of other barbiturates whose pK_a values lie outside the appropriate range[26]. Forced acidic diuresis increases the excretion of amphetamine[3, 9] and pethidine[4].

The over-all elimination rate constant (k_{el}) of a drug is equal to the sum of the individual rate constants of metabolism (k_{met}) and excretion (k_{exc}) (see Chapter 2). Thus:

$$k_{el} = k_{met} + k_{exc}$$

From this equation it is apparent that for drugs whose k_{met} is large in comparison to their k_{exc}, alterations in renal function can produce little pharmacokinetic change. Thus the elimination rate of paracetamol, which is normally excreted almost entirely as its glucuronide and sulphate (see Chapter 2), will not be influenced by even the most profound alterations in renal function. By contrast, for drugs whose k_{exc} is large compared with their k_{met} the converse holds, so that, for example, the elimination rate constant of benzylpenicillin which is normally about 1.4 hours^{-1} ($T_{\frac{1}{2}} = 0.5$ hours) is reduced to 0.07 hours^{-1} ($T_{\frac{1}{2}} = 10$ hours) in anuric patients. Alterations in renal function can therefore be expected to influence the elimination rate of only those drugs for which excretion by the kidney plays an important role.

An increase in penicillin clearance has been demonstrated in man[32] following the administration of bacterial pyrogens. The most likely explanation lies in the increased renal blood flow (without change in glomerular filtration rate) which occurs during fever[36], and which would be expected to enhance the elimination of drugs undergoing active tubular secretion. This possibility has, as yet, not been actively pursued.

Drugs in renal failure

Drug accumulation due to impaired renal excretion occurs in patients with intrinsic renal disease and in patients with poor renal perfusion (as in hypovolaemic shock). Furthermore, glomerular filtration rate is reduced in both the old and the very young, whilst tubular secretion is also impaired in the latter age-group[8]. In general, it can be shown that the elimination rate constant of most drugs declines linearly with falling glomerular filtration rate[11] *(Figure 8.3)*. It is therefore possible to predict the elimination rate constant of a drug in a patient with renal disease if the glomerular filtration is known and if data are available on the elimination rate constants for both normal and anephric subjects. Such information can be used to calculate both the loading and the maintenance doses required by patients with renal impairment[11]. The method is described in detail in Appendix A. Such calculations may, however, be of restricted value in clinical practice for two reasons: first, it is often necessary to start drug therapy before the creatinine clearance is known; secondly, profound changes in glomerular filtration rate frequently occur overnight in infected patients with renal failure which will invalidate the basis of the calculations. Monitoring of plasma concentrations (see Chapter 10) of potentially toxic drugs is therefore obligatory.

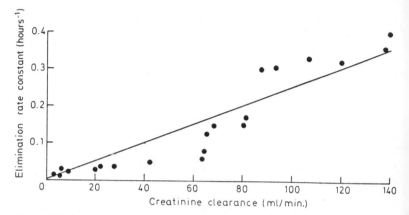

Figure 8.3. Relationship between the elimination rate constant of gentamicin and the endogenous creatinine clearance in patients with normal and diminished renal function. (Constructed from the data of Gyselynck, Forrey and Cutler, 1971[15])

An alternative approach is to adjust drug dosage purely on the basis of plasma creatinine concentrations[17]. No alteration in dosage schedules is necessary for patients with plasma creatinine concentrations below 3 mg/100 ml. Patients with plasma creatinine concentrations above this value are given the full normal loading dose which will produce the anticipated initial plasma concentration of drug. Maintenance doses of half the loading dose are given[20] at intervals which depend upon the plasma creatinine and the drug being used (see Appendix B). This method can readily be applied to the use of antibiotics, many of which accumulate in the presence of renal failure. These drugs are conveniently divided into four categories[25]. The first group, comprising those drugs which are excreted largely by the kidneys and which have a low therapeutic ratio, include the aminoglycosides and colistin; major reduction in the frequency of administration of maintenance doses, together with monitoring of blood levels, is necessary. Less drastic dosage reduction is needed during the administration of drugs in group II — benzylpenicillin, carbenicillin, cephalothin and cotrimoxazole — and no dosage reduction is required during administration of cloxacillin, erythromycin, novobiocin, fucidin, isoniazid and rifampicin (group III). Drugs in group IV (chloramphenicol, nitrofurantoin and the tetracyclines) should be avoided altogether because of toxicity in patients with renal disease. This method of dosage reduction, though simple to apply, suffers from two disadvantages. First, plasma creatinine concentrations do not necessarily reflect the degree of renal impairment, and secondly, drug administration in this way tends to produce large swings in plasma concentrations which may be undesirable.

Patients with renal impairment are especially prone to toxicity from cardiac glycosides, partly because these drugs undergo renal excretion and are therefore retained and partly because of the disturbances in potassium homoeostasis that so frequently occur in such patients. Since phenothiazines used as antipruritics and antiemetics and their metabolites undergo partial renal elimination, accumulation in patients with renal disease can produce oculogyric crises that may be confused with uraemic fits[19].

Patients with poor renal function may accumulate metabolites of those drugs whose principal elimination is via metabolism. Chloramphenicol glucuronide[22] and acetylsulphamethoxazole[7] have been shown to accumulate in this manner. Although this process is potentially hazardous, little information on its importance is as yet available. The influence of renal disease on drug distribution, metabolism and response is discussed in Chapters 4 and 7.

Biliary excretion

Certain drugs and drug metabolites are excreted by the liver cells into bile and pass into the intestine. The mechanisms involved are incompletely defined but experiments in animals indicate that separate transport systems exist for organic acids such as probenecid[14] and chlorothiazide[16], for organic bases[35] and for non-electrolytes such as ouabain[23]. Biliary excretion appears to be favoured by polar compounds of comparatively high molecular weight (more than 300) so that glucuronide conjugates of many drugs are handled in this manner. Thus, 80 per cent of an oral dose of carbenoxolone in man can be recovered from bile as the glucuronide[30].

Drugs which are secreted into bile pass into the intestine, from which reabsorption may take place (see Chapter 3). Such enterohepatic circulation can have a marked effect on drug pharmacokinetics. In normal rats, for example, glutethimide has a half-life of 24 hours but in animals with biliary fistulae this is reduced to 6 hours[18]. Gut bacteria (see Chapter 3) appear to play an important role in the enterohepatic circulation of compounds excreted in bile as glucuronides.

Thus, stilboestrol is extensively excreted in rat bile as stilboestrol monoglucuronide which is not reabsorbed. However, bacterial beta-glucuronidase in the intestinal lumen yields stilboestrol which is available for reabsorption. The importance of these mechanisms in man (and the influence of disease thereon) is largely unexplored and the extreme degree of interspecies variability[1] makes extrapolation from animal data unwarranted. Those studies which have been undertaken in man have been largely concerned with estimating antibiotic concentrations in hepatic and gall-bladder bile in order to establish rational therapeutic principles in the management of biliary tract infections. Two sharply divisible classes have emerged: sulphonamides, chloramphenicol[13], streptomycin[45], kanamycin[31], gentamicin[38] and cephalexin are excreted in low concentration, usually less than that occurring in blood; penicillin[45], ampicillin[6], tetracyclines[21] and rifamycin[2] are excreted in high concentration. In patients with cystic or common bile duct obstruction, biliary concentrations of ampicillin are considerably reduced[29]. Gall-bladder bile concentrations of antibiotics are higher than hepatic bile[33, 44] in patients with radiologically functional gall bladders. Patients with non-functioning gall bladders have considerably lower concentrations. It should be emphasized, however, that antibiotics which are not concentrated in bile may yet be valuable chemotherapeutic agents in eradicating infections of the biliary tree if the organisms responsible are sufficiently sensitive.

Other routes of excretion

Drugs are present in saliva, sweat, milk, lacrimal and vaginal secretions largely on the basis of non-ionic diffusion[39]. These routes are quantitatively unimportant in drug excretion and are not a source of variability in human drug response. The secretion of basic drugs into the gastric lumen (where the pH is low) offers a method by which such drugs are made re-available for absorption. Recycling in this way, however, is unlikely to be of sufficient magnitude as to be an important source of variability in man. Mammary secretion may be responsible for the transfer of drugs from mother to baby, producing unwanted effects in the latter.

References

1. Abou-El-Makarem, M. M., Millburn, P., Smith, R. L. and Williams, R. T. (1967). 'Biliary excretion of foreign compounds: species differences in biliary excretion.' *Biochem. J.* **105**, 1289–1293

2. Acocella, G., Mattiussi, R., Nicolis, F. B., Pallanza, R. and Tenconi, L. T. (1968). 'Biliary excretion of antibiotics in man.' *Gut* 9, 536–545
3. Asatoor, A. M., Galman, B. R., Johnson, J. R. and Milne, M. D. (1965). 'The excretion of dexamphetamine and its derivatives.' *Br. J. Pharmac.* 24, 293–300
4. Asatoor, A. M., London, D. R., Milne, M. D. and Simenhoff, M. L. (1963). 'The excretion of pethidine and its derivatives.' *Br. J. Pharmac.* 20, 285–298
5. Asatoor, A. M., and Milne, M. D. (1965). Unpublished observations quoted in *Fundamentals of Drug Metabolism and Drug Disposition.* Ed. by B. N. La Du, H. G. Mandel and E. L. Way. (1971). Baltimore, Md: Williams & Wilkins
6. Ayliffe, G. A. J. and Davies, A. (1965). 'Ampicillin levels in human bile.' *Br. J. Pharmac.* 24, 189–193
7. Baithke, R., Golde, G. and Gahl, G. (1972). 'Sulphamethoxazole/trimethoprim: pharmacokinetic studies in patients with chronic renal failure.' *Eur. J. clin. Pharmac.* 4, 233–240
8. Barnett, H. L. (1950). 'Kidney function in young infants.' *Pediatrics, Springfield* 5, 171–179
9. Beckett, A. H. M., Rowland, M. and Turner, P. (1965). 'The influence of urinary pH on excretion of amphetamine.' *Lancet* 1, 303–305
10. Dettli, L. and Spring, P. (1966). In *Physico-Chemical Aspects of Drug Action,* Vol. 7, pp. 5–37. Ed. by E. J. Ariëns. Oxford: Pergamon
11. Dettli, L., Spring, P. and Ryter, S. (1971). 'Multiple dose kinetics and drug dosage in patients with kidney disease.' *Acta Pharmac. Tox.* 29 (Suppl. 3), 211–224
12. Field, J. B., Ohta, M., Boyle, C. and Remer, A. (1967). 'Potentiation of acetohexamide hypoglycaemia by phenylbutazone.' *New Engl. J. Med.* 277, 889–894
13. Garrod, L. P. and O'Grady, F. (1971). *Antibiotic and Chemotherapy,* 3rd ed. Edinburgh and London: Churchill Livingstone
14. Guarino, A. M. and Schanker, L. S. (1968). 'Biliary excretion of probenecid and its glucuronides.' *J. Pharmac. exp. Ther.* 164, 387–395
15. Gyselynck, A-M., Forrey, A. and Cutler, R. (1971). 'Pharmacokinetics of gentamicin distribution and plasma and renal clearance.' *J. infect. Dis.* 124, S70–76
16. Hart, L. G. and Schanker, L. S. (1966). 'Active transport of chlorothiazide into bile.' *Am. J. Physiol.* 211, 643–646
17. Jones, N. F. and Wing, A. J. (1971). 'Renal disease.' In *A Guide to the Therapy of Common Diseases,* pp. 25–54. Ed. by W. I. Cranston. Lancaster: Medical and Technical Publ.
18. Keberle, H., Hoffmann, K. and Bernhard, K. (1962). 'The metabolism of glutethimide (Doriden).' *Experientia* 18, 105–111

19. Kerr, D. N. S. and Walls, J. (1970) 'Medication in renal failure.' *Prescrib. J.* **10**, 118–124

20. Kunin, C. M. (1967). 'A guide to use of antibiotics in patients with renal disease. A table of recommended doses and factors governing serum levels.' *Ann. intern. Med.* **67**, 151–158

21. Kunin, C. M. and Finland, M. (1959). 'Restrictions imposed on antibiotic therapy by renal failure.' *Archs intern. Med.* **104**, 1030–1050

22. Kunin, C. M., Glazko, A. J. and Finland, M. (1959). 'Persistence of antibiotics in blood of patients with acute renal failure. II. Chloramphenicol and its metabolic products in the blood of patients with severe renal disease or hepatic cirrhosis.' *J. clin. Invest.* **38**, 1498–1508

23. Kupferberg, H. J. and Schanker, L. S. (1968). 'Biliary excretion of ouabain-^{3}H and its uptake by liver slices in the rat.' *Am. J. Physiol.* **214**, 1048–1053

24. Lawson, A. A. H., Proudfoot, A. T., Brown, S. S., MacDonald, R. H., Fraser, A. G., Cameron, J. C. and Matthew, H. (1969). 'Forced diuresis in the treatment of acute salicylate poisoning in adults.' *Q. Jl Med.* **38**(NS), 31–48

25. Leading Article (1971). 'Antibacterial agents in renal failure.' *Br. med. J.* **1**, 621–622

26. Linton, A. L., Luke, R. G. and Briggs, J. D. (1967). 'Methods of forced diuresis and its application in barbiturate poisoning.' *Lancet* **2**, 377–380

27. Milne, M. D., Scribner, B. H. and Crawford, M. A. (1958). 'Nonionic diffusion and the excretion of weak acids and bases.' *Am. J. Med.* **24**, 709–729

28. Morgan, A. G. and Polak, A. (1971). 'The excretion of salicylate in salicylate poisoning.' *Clin. Sci.* **41**, 475–484

29. Mortimer, P. R., Mackie, D. B. and Haynes, S. (1969). 'Ampicillin levels in human bile in the presence of biliary tract disease.' *Br. med. J.* **3**, 88–89

30. Parke, D. V., Humphrey, M. J., Chakraborty, J. and Lindup, W. E. (1972). 'Biochemical pharmacology of carbenoxolone.' *Proc. 5th Int. Congr. Pharmacol.*, p. 176. Basle: Karger

31. Preston, F. W., Silverman, M., Henegar, C. C. and Neveril, E. (1960). 'The excretion of kanamycin in bile and pancreatic fluid.' *Antibiotics A.* **7**, 857–861

32. Rantz, L. A. and Kirby, W. M. M. (1944). 'The absorption and excretion of penicillin following continuous intravenous and subcutaneous administration.' *J. clin. Invest.* **23**, 789–794

33. Sales, J. E. L., Sutcliffe, M. and O'Grady, F. (1972). 'Cephalexin levels in human bile in presence of biliary tract disease.' *Br. med. J.* **3**, 441–443

34. Schachter, D. and Manis, J. G. (1958). 'Salicylate and salicyl conjugates: fluorimetric estimation, biosynthesis and renal excretion in man.' *J. clin. Invest.* **37**, 800–807

35. Schanker, L. S. and Solomon, H. M. (1963). 'Active transport of quaternary ammonium compounds into bile.' *Am. J. Physiol.* **204**, 829–832

36. Smith, H. W. (1956). *Principles of Renal Physiology*. New York: Oxford University Press

37. Smith, P. K., Gleason, H. L., Stoll, C. G. and Ogorzalek, S. (1946). 'Studies on the pharmacology of salicylates'. *J. Pharmac. exp. Ther.* **87**, 237–255

38. Smithivas, T., Hyams, P. J. and Rahal, J. J. (1971). 'Gentamicin and ampicillin levels in human bile'. *J. infect. Dis.* **124**, S106–108

39. Stowe, C. M. and Plaa, G. L. (1968). 'Extrarenal excretion of drugs and chemicals.' *A. Rev. Pharmacol.* **8**, 337–356

40. Volle, R. L., Green, R. E. and Peters, L. (1960). 'Renal tubular transport relationships between N^1-methylnicotinamide (NMN), mecamylamine, quinine, quinidine and quinacrine in the avian kidney.' *J. Pharmac. exp. Ther.* **129**, 388–393

41. Watrous, W. M., May, D. G. and Fujimoto, J. M. (1970). 'Mechanism of the renal tubular transport of morphine and morphine ethereal sulphate.' *J. Pharmac. exp. Ther.* **172**, 224–229

42. Woodbury, D. M. (1970). 'Analgesic–antipyretics, anti-inflammatory agents and inhibitors of uric acid synthesis.' In *The Pharmacological Basis of Therapeutics*, 4th edn., pp. 314–347. Ed. by L. S. Goodman and A. Gilman. New York and London: Collier-Macmillan

43. Yü, T. F. and Guttman, A. B. (1955). 'Paradoxical retention of uric acid by uricosuric agents in low dosage.' *Proc. Soc. exp. Biol. Med.* **90**, 542–547

44. Zaslow, J., Counseller, V. S. and Hillman, F. R. (1947). 'The excretion and concentration of penicillin and streptomycin in the abnormal human biliary tract. I. Gall bladder.' *Surg. Gynec. Obstet.* **84**, 16–20

45. Zaslow, J., Counseller, V. S. and Hillman, F. R. (1947). 'The excretion and concentration of penicillin and streptomycin in the abnormal human biliary tract. II. Hepatic bile.' *Surg. Gynec. Obstet.* **84**, 140–152

CHAPTER 9

Tissue Sensitivity

It is apparent from investigations discussed in previous chapters that most variability in the clinical response to drugs is pharmacokinetic in origin. The tissues of the body respond differently because they contain different concentrations of drug. There remains, however, some variability in drug response which appears to arise independently of pharmacokinetic factors. By implication, tissues respond differently because of intrinsic differences in their sensitivity to particular drug actions. Such differences may be quantitative or qualitative. The latter result in abnormal clinical responses and are readily explicable in terms of abnormalities of tissue enzyme content. A few common examples are discussed in this chapter.

Quantitative differences in response are less readily understood. Animal work reveals remarkable conformity in the behaviour of receptors between different individuals and even between species, although, as mentioned elsewhere, the conditions employed in their study are tightly controlled. On the other hand, in the peripheral nervous system at least, receptor sensitivity can be altered. Physical or pharmacological denervation, for example, may cause supersensitivity. This is well illustrated by the exaggerated reactions of guanethidine-treated animals and patients to sympathomimetic agents. By contrast, repeated large doses of drugs may cause desensitization, a phenomenon which may help to explain the tolerance which is developed by drug addicts. In the absence of such treatments, however, interindividual differences in sensitivity must be taken to indicate the presence of different numbers or varieties of receptors or differences in the ways in which such receptors initiate tissue responses. Unfortunately, information on such matters is almost entirely lacking, although a number of observations indicate that the differences may be at least partly genetic in origin.

Quantitative differences in drug response

Taste sensitivity

Perhaps the best documented examples of variability in tissue response are those of taste thresholds to quinine[19] and phenylthiourea (PTC)[4], probably because they are readily measured. Sensitivity to the taste of quinine is distributed normally in the population *(Figure 9.1a)*, but that of PTC is bimodal *(Figure 9.1b)*, being subject to a genetic polymorphism, the greater sensitivity being inherited as a dominant character. Smell thresholds are also subject to considerable individual variability[7].

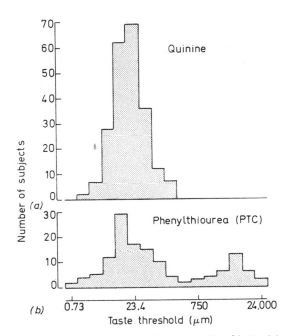

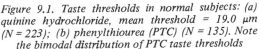

Figure 9.1. Taste thresholds in normal subjects: (a) quinine hydrochloride, mean threshold = 19.0 μm (N = 223); (b) phenylthiourea (PTC) (N = 135). Note the bimodal distribution of PTC taste thresholds

Although phenomena are of little clinical significance in themselves, some recent work suggests that associations may exist between sensitivities of receptors in taste buds and those which determine responses in the central and peripheral autonomic nervous systems. Thus Knopp and his colleagues[23] have reported that patients who are most sensitive to the extrapyramidal effects of trifluoperazine have significantly lower taste thresholds to quinine. These results are of particular interest in the light of the knowledge that a hereditary predisposition is involved in drug-induced parkinsonism[30]. A similar finding involving the action of hyoscine N-butylbromide on the autonomic nervous system has been reported by Joyce, Pan and Varonos[22]. They have shown significant correlations between taste sensitivity and responses of the heart and salivary glands to this drug. The implication of this evidence is that individuals may have preset sensitivities in a variety of tissues to the effect of drugs and that these determine the responses of the tissues to drug administration. Comparative studies of the most sensitive and the least sensitive individuals, as detected by taste threshold measurements, suggest that there may be personality and behavioural differences involved in the sensitivity pattern[15].

The hope has been expressed[22] that measurement of taste sensitivity might have value in the prediction of the intensity of systemic drug response. An unpublished investigation by the authors of the relationship between taste threshold and intensity of heart rate change following intramuscular atropine (similar to that described by Joyce, Pan and Varonos[22]) reveals that this is unlikely. Although it confirms the significant relationship between the two, it shows also that only 20 per cent of the variability in heart rate response is accountable on the basis of taste threshold differences. It is therefore unlikely that there would be clinical value in the measurement of individual taste thresholds.

Mydriatic drugs

Marked differences in response are seen also after local instillation of ephedrine and other mydriatics into the eye, at least partly in association with differing amounts of iris pigmentation[21, 32], which are presumably genetic in origin. The reason for the well recognized failure of darkly pigmented irides to respond to almost any mydriatic is not clear but it may be due to an excess of parasympathetic over sympathetic tone. An enzyme study of animal eyes[1] revealed that pigmented irides had more dopa oxidase than had non-pigmented irides. This suggests that in the former there may be a relative shortage of sympathetic transmitter because dopa (the precursor) is preferentially metabolized into the pigment pathway. Other explanations for the failure of drugs to influence darkly pigmented irides are failure of penetration[20] and preferential binding to the pigment[35]. This subject clearly needs further investigation. Twin experiments by Bertler and Smith[3] revealed remarkably great apparent genetic influences on pupil size and its response to phenylephrine, even in blue-eyed subjects, and on the heart rate and its response to hyoscine N-butylbromide. The results suggest that drug responses of the eye and of the heart are partly determined by the levels of parasympathetic and sympathetic tone and that these levels are genetically influenced.

Anticoagulants

Variability in tissue response is thought to be involved in the rather rare finding of inherited resistance to anticoagulants reported by O'Reilly and his colleagues[33, 34]. Two families are described, many members of which require 20 or more times the usual dose and vastly greater plasma levels of coumarin anticoagulant for a reasonable clinical response. The disposition of warfarin in these subjects appears to be normal as judged by measurements of half-lives and protein binding. Human anticoagulant resistance of this type is therefore similar to that found in rats[11]. A lesser degree of variability is revealed also by recent studies of Breckenridge[5], who found that individual steady-state plasma concentrations of warfarin varied some sixfold among patients treated to the same degree of anticoagulation. The evidence of these observations is taken to indicate that the anticoagulant receptors or the enzyme mechanisms involved in clotting factor synthesis must vary greatly between individuals in showing different degrees of susceptibility to the drug. The interpretation of these findings is, however, uncertain because of the competitive nature of the drug involved. Similar findings could result from variability in the amount of vitamin K_1 available to the liver of these individuals. In the case of the rare familial resistance, however, vitamin K_1 availability cannot be grossly abnormal because the individuals are known to respond normally to its administration.

The anticoagulant effects of dicoumarol and warfarin can be increased clinically by the concurrent administration of D-thyroxine, clofibrate or norethandrolone (an anabolic steroid). Given over two weeks, these drugs do not influence metabolism of the anticoagulant[38] as do other drugs discussed in Chapter 7. A detailed analysis of the effect of D-thyroxine suggests that it increases the affinity of the anticoagulant for its hepatic receptor site[40], a novel type of drug interaction which merits further study. The mode of action, however, is not certain because exactly similar effects (potentiation without change in metabolic breakdown) could arise from a combination of impaired protein binding with slight inhibition of metabolism, or from reduced availability of vitamin K_1. With clofibrate at least the first of these possibilities is quite likely (see Chapters 4 and 7).

Psychotropic drugs

Beneficial effects of drug treatment, especially in the management of psychiatric illness, are often ascribed to the patient's genetic make-up. Thus theories have been raised that relate inheritance and good response to MAO inhibitor or tricyclic antidepressant administration. From present evidence it seems likely that beneficial results of such therapy are related most directly to pharmacokinetic handling of the drug and to the nature of the illness being treated[27]. To the extent that both these are subject to genetic influence, the drug effects must also be so influenced. The factors involved are discussed in detail by Angst[2].

Abnormal drug responses

Glucose-6-phosphate dehydrogenase deficiency

Inherited enzyme abnormalities are known to influence the duration of drug action by effects exerted on the drug's own metabolism (see Chapter 6). Abnormal responses to drug administration occur also because of enzyme abnormalities in the tissues. The best known of these is erythrocyte glucose-6-phosphate dehydrogenase (G-6-PD) deficiency, which occurs quite frequently among coloured peoples of Africa and the USA, among some Mediterraneans, Kurdish and Iraqi Jews and among Filipinos. In Caucasians it is very rare. The lesion is associated with a chronic deficit of reduced thiol (−SH) groups in erythrocytes and probably an accumulation of oxidized glutathione (glutathione disulphide). This accumulation is thought to confer on the individual the selective survival advantage against falciparum malaria infection[24] which causes persistence of the enzyme abnormality in areas of endemic malarial infection[29]. The condition is inherited but the mode of inheritance is complex, there being a number of different factors involved. Oxidation of the few reduced thiol groups in the erythrocytes by drugs causes acute haemolysis, particularly among older cells. Younger cells, however, are not usually affected so that the incident of haemolysis is usually transient. An account of the biochemical mechanisms involved was given by Carson[8], and of the clinical implications by Prankerd[37]. Any drug which is an oxidizing agent and a number of others may precipitate haemolytic episodes in G-6-PD deficient subjects. The abnormality is sometimes called primaquine sensitivity because the first observations were made with this drug. Many others have the same effect; a list of the most important ones is given in Table 9.1.

TABLE 9.1. Drugs which cause Haemolysis in Glucose-6-phosphate Dehydrogenase Deficiency

8-Aminoquinolines	Pamaquin, pentaquine, primaquine, quinocide
Sulphonamides and sulphones	Sulphacetamide, sulphafurazole, sulphamethoxy-pyridazine, sulphanilamide, sulphapyridine, sulphasalazine, dapsone
Nitrofurans	Furazolidone, nitrofurantoin, nitrofurazone
Analgesics	Amidopyrine, antipyrine (phenazone), aspirin, phenacetin
Others	Acetylphenylhydrazine, chloramphenicol, para-aminosalicylate (PAS), probenecid, quinidine, quinine

From Marks and Banks, 1965[25]

Hereditary methaemoglobinaemia

In the various types of hereditary methaemoglobinaemia involving NADP-diaphorase deficiency[39] or methaemoglobin reductase deficiency[9], the administration of drugs which are oxidizing agents causes an increase in methaemoglobinaemia. Nitrites show this effect markedly but any of the drugs listed in Table 9.1 could do the same thing.

The occurrence of methaemoglobinaemia following drug administration is not, however, restricted to people with this disorder. Cowan and Evans[10] showed that primaquine administration caused methaemoglobinaemia in most of a group of 59 normal subjects and that the concentration produced was roughly normally distributed. The production of overt methaemoglobinaemia may therefore be merely an exaggeration of the normal response.

Porphyria

Abnormal responses to drugs occur also in the hepatic porphyrias, probably in association with increases in hepatic delta-aminolaevulinic acid synthetase (ALA synthetase), activity of which is already abnormally high in these conditions[28, 31]. The relevance to this discussion lies in the fact that most of the drugs which precipitate overt attacks of porphyrinuria are known to be enzyme inducers (Chapter 7). In a detailed discussion of the causes of hepatic porphyrias and of the effects of drugs, Granick[18] has proposed that the activity of ALA synthetase is normally repressed by haem. He suggests that the disease is caused by a variation in an operator gene which is poorly responsive to the normal repressor. Inducing agents are thought to precipitate the condition by removal of the repressor. A general review of the effects of drugs on porphyrin metabolism is given by Matteis[26].

Attacks of porphyria can be precipitated by many different drugs (Table 9.2), the most important of which are the barbiturates and other hypnotic drugs, anticonvulsants and ethanol, oral hypoglycaemic agents and hormones. Oral contraceptive agents can cause exacerbations but they have also been found in some cases to ameliorate attacks associated with menstruation[36]. It is apparent that sensitivities of patients with acute intermittent porphyria to barbiturates and other drugs vary widely, some developing serious symptoms after single doses, others requiring prolonged administration of quite large doses before developing an attack[17]. The failure of porphyric subjects to show sensitivity to single doses, as in the family from Jutland described by With[41], is therefore of little significance.

TABLE 9.2. Drugs which Precipitate Attacks of Acute Porphyria in Man

Hypnotics and tranquillizers	Barbiturates, chlordiazepoxide, dichloralphenazone, glutethimide, meprobamate
Anticonvulsants	Ethosuximide, methsuximide, phensuximide, phenytoin
Hypoglycaemic agents	Chlorpropamide, tolbutamide
Others	Aminopyrine, ethanol, griseofulvin, sulphonamides, sex hormones, oral contraceptives

From Matteis, 1967[26] © Williams & Wilkins Co.

Malignant hyperpyrexia

The well recognized condition of malignant hyperpyrexia occurs as a rare complication of general anaesthesia. Following the administration of an inhalational anaesthetic, most often halothane, and usually of suxamethonium as well, there is increasing muscle stiffness and hyperpyrexia. Some cases appear to be hereditary in origin and others sporadic[6, 14]. During the episode there is progressive muscle damage and consequent high serum levels of creatine phosphokinase, phosphate and potassium[13] and acidosis. Close relatives of hereditary cases show evidence of myopathy, associated with raised serum levels of creatine phosphokinase and aspartate aminotransferase[12]. The exact cause of the condition is uncertain and probably differs between individuals affected. In some cases, muscle stiffness may result from undue calcium permeability of the sarcoplasmic membrane, induced by anaesthetics. In others, a similar disturbance involving the mitochondrial membrane may increase heat production[16].

References

1. Angenent, W. J. and Koelle, G. B. (1953). 'A possible enzymatic basis for the differential action of mydriatics on light and dark irides.' *J. Physiol. Lond.* **119**, 102–117
2. Angst, J. (1964). 'Antidepressiver Effekt und genetische Faktoren.' *Arzneimittel-Forsch.* **14**, 496–500
3. Bertler, Å. and Smith, S. E. (1971). 'Genetic influences in drug responses of the eye and the heart.' *Clin. Sci.* **40**, 403–410
4. Blakeslee, A. F. and Salmon, M. R. (1931). 'Odor and taste blindness.' *Eugenl News* **16**, 105
5. Breckenridge, A. (1972). Personal communication
6. Britt, B. A., Locher, W. G. and Kalow, W. (1969). 'Hereditary aspects of malignant hyperthermia.' *Can. Anaesth. Soc. J.* **16**, 89–98
7. Brown, K. S., MacLean, C. M. and Robinette, R. R. (1968). 'The distribution of the sensitivity to chemical odors in man.' *Hum. Biol.* **40**, 456–472
8. Carson, P. E. (1960). 'Glucose-6-phosphate dehydrogenase deficiency in hemolytic anemia.' *Fedn Proc.* **19**, 995–1006
9. Cawein, M., Behlen, C. H., Lappat, E. J. and Cohn, J. E. (1964). 'Hereditary diaphorase deficiency and methemoglobinemia.' *Archs intern. Med.* **113**, 578–585
10. Cowan, W. K. and Evans, D. A. P. (1964). 'Primaquine and methemoglobin.' *Clin. Pharmac. Ther.* **5**, 307–309
11. Davis, R. J. and Davies, B. H. (1970). 'The biochemistry of warfarin resistance in the rat.' *Biochem. J.* **118**, 44P–45P
12. Denborough, M. A., Ebeling, P., King, J. O. and Zapf, P. (1970). 'Myopathy and malignant hyperpyrexia.' *Lancet* **1**, 1138–1140
13. Denborough, M. A., Forster, J. F. A., Hudson, M. C., Carter, N. G. and Zapf, P. (1970). 'Biochemical changes in malignant hyperpyrexia.' *Lancet* **1**, 1137–1138
14. Denborough, M. A. and Lovell, R. R. H. (1960). 'Anaesthetic deaths in a family.' *Lancet* **2**, 45

15. Fischer, R. (1971). 'Gustatory, behavioral and pharmacological manifestations of chemoreception in man.' In *Gustation and Olfaction*, pp. 187—235. Ed. by G. Ohloff and A. F. Thomas. London: Academic

16. Furniss, P. (1971). 'The aetiology of malignant hyperpyrexia.' *Proc. R. Soc. Med.* **64**, 216—220

17. Goldberg, A. (1959). 'Acute intermittent porphyria. A study of 50 cases.' *Q. Jl Med.* **28**, 183—209

18. Granick, S. (1966). 'The induction in vitro of the synthesis of δ-aminolevulinic acid synthetase in chemical porphyria: a response to certain drugs, sex hormones, and foreign chemicals.' *J. biol. Chem.* **241**, 1359—1375

19. Hänig, D. P. (1901). 'Zur Psychophysik des Geschmackssinnes.' *Philos. Stud., Wundt.* **17**, 576—623

20. Harris, L. S. and Galin, M. A. (1971). 'Effect of ocular pigmentation on hypotensive response to pilocarpine.' *Am. J. Ophthal.* **72**, 923—925

21. Howard, H. J. and Lee, T. P. (1927). 'The effect of instillations of ephedrine solutions upon the eye.' *Proc. Soc. exp. Biol. Med.* **24**, 700—702

22. Joyce, C. R. B., Pan, L. and Varonos, D. D. (1968). 'Taste sensitivity may be used to predict pharmacological effects.' *Life Sci.* **7**, 533—537

23. Knopp, W., Fischer, R., Beck, J. and Teitelbaum, A. (1966). 'Clinical implications of the relation between taste sensitivity and the appearance of extrapyramidal side effects.' *Dis. nerv. Syst.* **27**, 729—735

24. Kosower, N. S. and Kosower, E. M. (1970). 'Molecular basis for selective advantage of glucose-6-phosphate-dehydrogenase-deficient individuals exposed to malaria.' *Lancet* **2**, 1343—1345

25. Marks, P. A. and Banks, J. (1965). 'Drug-induced hemolytic anemias associated with glucose-6-phosphate dehydrogenase deficiency: a genetically heterogeneous trait.' *Ann. N.Y. Acad. Sci.* **123**, 198—206

26. Matteis, F. de (1967). 'Disturbances of liver porphyrin metabolism caused by drugs.' *Pharmac. Rev.* **19**, 523—557

27. Mendlewicz, J., Fieve, R. R., Stallone, F. and Fleiss, J. L. (1972). 'Genetic history as a predictor of lithium response in manic-depressive illness.' *Lancet* **1**, 599—600

28. Moore, M. R., Turnbull, A. L., Barnardo, D., Beattie, A. D., Magnus, I. A. and Goldberg, A. (1972). 'Hepatic δ-aminolaevulinic acid synthetase activity in porphyria cutanea tarda.' *Lancet* **2**, 97—100

29. Motulsky, A. G. (1960). 'Metabolic polymorphisms and the role of infectious diseases in human evolution.' *Hum. Biol.* **32**, 28—62

30. Myrianthopoulos, N. C., Kurland, A. A. and Kurland, L. T. (1962). 'Hereditary predisposition in drug-induced parkinsonism.' *Archs Neurol. Chicago* **6**, 5—9

31. Nakao, K., Wada, O., Kitamura, T., Uono, K. and Urata, G. (1966). 'Activity of aminolevulinic acid synthetase in normal and porphyric human livers.' *Nature, Lond.* **210**, 838–839

32. Obianwu, H. O. and Rand, M. J. (1965). 'The relationship between the mydriatic action of ephedrine and the colour of the iris.' *Br. J. Ophthal.* **49**, 264–270

33. O'Reilly, R. A. (1970). 'The second reported kindred with hereditary resistance to oral anticoagulant drugs.' *New Engl. J. Med.* **282**, 1448–1451

34. O'Reilly, R. A., Aggeler, P. M., Hoag, M. S., Leong, L. S. and Kropatkin, M. L. (1964). 'Hereditary transmission of exceptional resistance to coumarin anticoagulant drugs. The first reported kindred.' *New Engl. J. Med.* **271**, 809–815

35. Patil, P. N. (1972). 'Cocaine-binding by the pigmented and the nonpigmented iris and its relevance to the mydriatic effect.' *Invest. Ophthalmol.* **11**, 739–746

36. Perlroth, M. G., Marver, H. S. and Tschudy, D. P. (1965). 'Oral contraceptive agents and the management of acute intermittent porphyria.' *J. Am. med. Ass.* **194**, 1037–1042

37. Prankerd, T. A. J. (1964). 'Glucose-6-phosphate dehydrogenase deficiency.' *Proc. R. Soc. Med.* **57**, 506–508

38. Schrogie, J. J. and Solomon, H. M. (1967). 'The anticoagulant response to bishydroxycoumarin. II. The effect of D-thyroxine, clofibrate and norethandrolone.' *Clin. Pharmac. Ther.* **8**, 70–77

39. Scott, E. M. (1960). 'The relation of diaphorase of human erythrocytes to inheritance of methemoglobinemia.' *J. clin. Invest.* **39**, 1176–1179

40. Solomon, H. M. and Schrogie, J. J. (1967). 'Change in receptor site affinity: a proposed explanation for the potentiating effect of D-thyroxine on the anticoagulant response to warfarin.' *Clin. Pharmac. Ther.* **8**, 797–799

41. With, T. K. (1965). 'Porphyria.' *Lancet* **1**, 916–917

CHAPTER 10

Monitoring Drug Therapy

Previous chapters have emphasized the difficulties inherent in predicting the effect of drug administration in an individual patient. Genetic and environmental influences, disease and the concomitant administration of other drugs all combine in determining the responses of such an individual to any therapeutic manoeuvre. The monitoring of drug therapy is therefore mandatory. This can be achieved either by monitoring drug effects or by monitoring the plasma levels of drugs. The two methods are not mutually exclusive.

Monitoring of drug effects

The traditional manner of monitoring drug therapy is to relate the dose to the pharmacological or therapeutic response. This method is valuable in certain instances, as for example in determining the dosage of thiopentone required for induction of anaesthesia. Useful information can be gained by questioning epileptic patients about the frequency of fits during the administration of antiepileptic drugs, whilst measurements of heart rate and blood pressure are of value in determining dosage regimens of cardiac glycosides and hypotensive agents respectively. The monitoring of drugs with a low therapeutic ratio has involved the use of more sophisticated tests of pharmacological effects. Oral anticoagulant therapy is now universally adjusted by measuring the hypoprothrombinaemic response[39]. The rosette inhibition test[38] appears to be of value in determining immunosuppressive drug dosage after renal transplantation[10], whilst the inhibition of rubidium-86 uptake by the red blood cells of digitalized patients may prove to be a good indication of the pharmacological (biochemical) effect of cardiac glycosides[27].

Monitoring of plasma levels — a pharmacokinetic approach

It is apparent that, whilst monitoring by pharmacological or therapeutic response is suitable for controlling the dosage of many drugs, there are clinical situations in which this is inappropriate, useless or even dangerously misleading. An alternative method of monitoring drug therapy is by measuring plasma concentrations of drugs. On theoretical grounds this is likely to be useful only if the following conditions are satisfied.

(1)   There must be a relatively constant interindividual relationship between the concentration of the drug in the plasma and at its site of action. In practice, this can rarely be determined directly.

(2)   The drug should act reversibly because the effects of irreversibly acting drugs (such as reserpine and MAO inhibitors) persist for long periods after the agent has been eliminated from the plasma.

(3)   The drug itself (and not a metabolite) should be the mediator of the pharmacological and therapeutic effects. Alternatively, the active metabolite itself should be measured.

With these factors in mind, measurements of plasma levels of drugs would be expected to be of clinical value:

(1)   with drugs whose steady-state plasma concentrations show wide interindividual differences;

(2)   with drugs of low therapeutic ratio;

(3)   with drugs for which the clinical distinction between overdosage and underdosage is difficult or impossible;

(4)   during the simultaneous administration of several drugs when serious interactions might be anticipated;

(5)   in patients with renal impairment, for drugs whose major route of elimination is via the kidneys;

(6)   in patients with liver disease, for drugs whose major route of elimination is via hepatic metabolism;

(7)   where there is doubt as to whether the drugs prescribed are actually being taken.

Although this aspect of clinical pharmacology is at an early stage, there are a number of drugs whose toxic and therapeutic effects correlate well with plasma concentrations. The clinical interpretation of data on plasma levels in individual patients is, however, valueless unless the following factors are taken into account. First, steady-state plasma concentrations of a drug which is given by repetitive dosing (without a loading dose) will be reached only after about five half-lives (see Chapter 2); thus, for a drug with a half-life of three days, steady-state conditions will be achieved only after two weeks. Secondly, plasma sampling must be performed at a constant time after the last dose of the drug to avoid post-absorption peaks. The usual practice is to sample just prior to the next dose. This requirement is fundamental. If the timing of sampling is ignored, accurate assessment of further dose requirements is impossible and comparisons of results between different laboratories become meaningless. This has been particularly evident in recent publications concerning the pharmacokinetic handling of digoxin, equilibration of which in body tissues takes several hours to achieve. There is no doubt that standardization of sampling times between different laboratories would be of considerable value.

Antibiotics

The assay of plasma concentrations of antibiotics is now a routine investigation in many microbiological laboratories. There are three principal indications for such measurements. First, to verify that adequate plasma concentrations are being obtained when there is doubt as to the adequacy of gastrointestinal absorption. Secondly, to ascertain that bactericidal plasma concentrations are present in patients with septicaemia or subacute bacterial endocarditis. Concentrations in c.s.f. are of similar value in patients with meningitis. Thirdly, to ensure that toxic antibiotics (e.g. streptomycin, kanamycin, gentamicin, vancomycin and colistin) do not accumulate to dangerous levels in patients with renal impairment. In this situation such monitoring is mandatory.

It is important to appreciate that most clinical antibiotic assays are performed using a biological method. If the patient is therefore receiving (or has recently been given) a second antibiotic of whose presence the bacteriologist is unaware, the results will be beyond interpretation.

Drugs acting on the central nervous system

Considerable evidence has now accumulated to indicate that there is a clinically useful correlation between the steady-state plasma concentrations of several drugs influencing the central nervous system and their pharmacological or therapeutic effects. Those drugs which have been the subject of most study are antidepressant and antiepileptic agents.

Antidepressant drugs. – Studies in psychiatric patients[2, 14, 53] have revealed wide interindividual differences in steady-state plasma

134

concentrations of tricyclic antidepressant drugs. This is well illustrated by the thirtyfold range in plasma concentrations following the administration of nortriptyline *(Figure 10.1)*. These differences are principally (but not exclusively) due to variability in the rate at which the drugs are metabolized. High plasma levels are associated with subjective side-effects[2, 53].

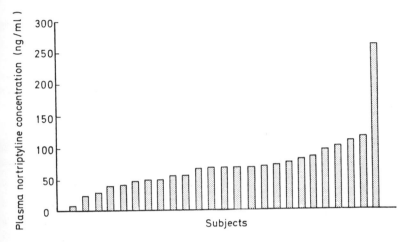

Figure 10.1. Steady-state plasma nortriptyline concentrations in 25 patients receiving 25 mg three times daily. Note the thirtyfold range in plasma levels. (From Sjöqvist, Hammer, Ideström, Lind, Tuck and Åsberg, 1968[44])

Of greater interest and importance is the apparent relationship found between the drug concentration and the antidepressant effect, as measured by a change in a depression rating scale following treatment. The study of Åsberg and her colleagues[3] using nortriptyline revealed a curved relationship, the therapeutic effect being optimal within a range of 50–139 ng/ml but slight at levels both below and above this range *(Figure 10.2)*. The poor response at low levels is due to the inadequate concentration of drug at the receptor; the failure to respond at high levels is less readily explicable but has been attributed to the alpha-adrenoceptor blocking action of the drug within the central nervous system. The clinical implications are, however, clear: only measurement of the plasma concentration can solve the dilemma of whether to increase or decrease the dose in a patient who has failed to respond satisfactorily. It should be emphasized that these findings only relate to patients with endogenous depression and not to reactive or neurotic depressives.

In other studies of such relationships using imipramine[53] and amitriptyline[14] good correlations have been found between plasma levels and therapeutic response. These investigations did not reveal poor responses at high levels as shown by the nortriptyline study. Whether

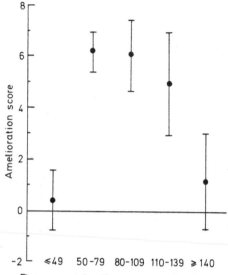

Figure 10.2. Relationship between amelioration of depressive symptoms and steady-state plasma concentrations in 39 patients receiving 25–75 mg nortriptyline three times daily. Note the curved relationship with optimal effects in the range 50–139 ng/ml. (From Åsberg, Cronholm, Sjöqvist and Tuck, 1971[3])

this represents a difference between the drugs used or merely that these latter investigations were performed with few patients in whom very high levels were not observed, is unclear. In both situations, interpretation of the results is complicated by the fact that the first metabolites are at least as active biologically as the parent drugs (desipramine as imipramine; nortriptyline as amitriptyline). The amitriptyline study revealed that the therapeutic effect was more closely correlated to the combined level of amitriptyline plus nortriptyline than to the level of either compound alone. Clearly, more detailed investigation is needed.

Antidepressant therapy is notoriously unsatisfactory in many patients. These studies provide at least part of the explanation of why this is so.

Lithium. – Treatment with lithium appears to be of value in the treatment of patients with both manic–depressive psychosis and recurrent depression[4, 21] provided that the plasma lithium concentration is maintained between 0.6 and 1.5 mEq/l. Perhaps surprisingly, the steady-state plasma lithium in volunteers receiving the same dose may vary from 0.45 to 1.34 mEq/l[43], the variability being due partly to differences in renal clearance and partly to differences in body build. The value of monitoring plasma lithium concentrations routinely has been underlined by the results of a study of 100 patients reputedly receiving the drug[23]; 34 patients had levels of less than 0.6 mEq/l, 8 had more than 2 mEq/l and in 10 patients lithium was undetectable.

Levodopa. – Monitoring plasma concentrations of levodopa in patients with Parkinson's disease does not appear to be of clinical value[1]. The therapeutic effect of this drug is mediated by the metabolite, dopamine, formed within the central nervous system, so that this finding is not necessarily surprising.

Phenytoin. – Clinical experience with the antiepileptic drug, phenytoin, has shown that with commonly used doses (300–400 mg daily in adults) the drug either abolishes or reduces the number of fits in the majority of patients. A minority, however, develop toxicity (nystagmus, ataxia and lethargy) at this dosage whilst a further group appear to derive no benefit. Phenytoin is eliminated predominantly by hepatic metabolism to para-hydroxyphenytoin (see Chapter 5) and, as would be expected, there are large interindividual differences in the steady-state concentration of the drug (see *Figure 5.1*). An apparent correlation exists between the steady-state plasma level of phenytoin and both its therapeutic[15, 34, 36] and toxic effects[13, 35]. Several investigations have confirmed that plasma levels of 10–20 μg/ml are required for effective seizure control. At plasma levels above 20 μg/ml side-effects occur and the severity of these is directly related to the plasma level *(Figure 10.3)*. With the advent of relatively simple gas-chromatographic methods for the estimation of phenytoin concentrations[6], occasional measurements in all patients taking the drug (particularly in those in whom seizure control is poor) are to be encouraged. It should be emphasized that all these concentrations refer to total plasma levels. Since phenytoin is 92 per cent bound to plasma proteins at therapeutic concentrations[37], only the unbound fraction in plasma is available for penetration into the central nervous system. The decreased binding of phenytoin in neonates[40] and uraemic patients[42] (see Chapter 4) explains why the drug produces seizure

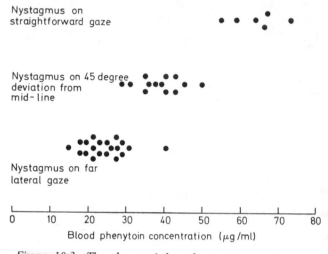

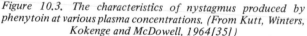

Figure 10.3. The characteristics of nystagmus produced by phenytoin at various plasma concentrations. (From Kutt, Winters, Kokenge and McDowell, 1964[35])

control in these two situations at very low plasma levels that are usually considered to be ineffective in adult epileptic patients with normal liver and kidney function[36]. The antiepileptic effect of phenobarbitone is also correlated with plasma concentrations of $10-20$ μg/ml[50]. However, since plasma concentrations of this drug vary only slightly between individual patients treated with the same dose, such monitoring is of much less value.

Drugs acting on the cardiovascular system

Lignocaine, procainamide, phenytoin and quinidine are all valuable drugs in the treatment of arrhythmias. For all four drugs there are considerable interindividual differences in the relationship between dosage and plasma concentration.

These differences are determined by variability in the various pharmacokinetic parameters discussed in previous chapters. Consideration of such parameters is important, and monitoring of plasma concentrations desirable, because for all four agents there appears to be a reasonable and clinically useful distinction between effective and toxic plasma levels (Table 10.1).

TABLE 10.1. Steady-state Plasma Concentrations (μg/ml) and Clinical Effects of Four Widely Used Antiarrhythmic Drugs

Clinical effect	Lignocaine	Procainamide	Phenytoin	Quinidine
Partially effective	1–2	2.5–4	5–10	1.5–3
Usually effective	2–5	4–10	10–20	3–6
Occasionally toxic	4–8	8–16	16–25	5–10
Usually toxic	>8	>16	>25	>10

From Koch-Weser, 1972[32]

Lignocaine. — Lignocaine is used extensively to suppress premature ventricular beats and in the treatment of ventricular tachyarrhythmias, particularly in patients with acute myocardial infarction[25]. Although in normal subjects prediction of the plasma level from the dose is reasonably reliable, this does not apply to patients with heart failure or liver disease. In the former, cardiac decompensation appears to be responsible for both a diminished volume of distribution and a fall in plasma clearance[51]. In the latter patients, plasma clearance is reduced due to diminished hepatic metabolism. Monitoring plasma levels to maintain effective, non-toxic concentrations is theoretically desirable but probably impractical in most centres because of the speed with which results need to be available if they are to have clinical value.

Procainamide. — Under normal dosage schedules, steady-state plasma levels of procainamide vary greatly between individuals, particularly in the presence of cardiac failure or renal insufficiency[31]. Low-output cardiac failure is associated with a reduction in its distribution volume (see Chapter 4), and impaired renal function reduces its most important mode of elimination. Both these conditions therefore predispose to elevated plasma levels if normal dosage schedules are followed. Since the useful therapeutic range of plasma concentration is strictly limited (4–8 μg/ml; see Table 10.1) and since toxicity involving mechanical and electrical disturbances in myocardial function appears at levels which are only slightly higher[33], there is obvious value in determining plasma concentrations. Particularly in the presence of cardiac or renal failure, but probably in all patients undergoing long-term procain-amide treatment monitoring of therapy to establish optimal dosage schedules is advisable.

Phenytoin. – The rationale for a pharmacokinetic approach to the use of phenytoin as an anticonvulsant agent is discussed above, and the same considerations apply to its use as an antiarrhythmic agent both orally and parenterally. Furthermore, the same steady-state plasma levels (10–20 μg/ml) appear to be required[11] for optimal therapeutic results in both clinical situations.

Quinidine. – Plasma quinidine concentrations are poorly correlated with dosage under conditions of diminished cardiac output and renal insufficiency[32], and elimination of the drug via the kidneys is depen-dent on urinary pH (see Chapter 8). A therapeutic effect is observed when plasma levels are in the range 2–5 μg/ml and toxic effects usually occur when the plasma concentration is in excess of 8 μg/ml[20]. Similar considerations apply as in the case of other antiarrhythmic agents and monitoring of therapy is clearly helpful.

Digitalis. – Two methods are currently available for the estimation of plasma digoxin concentrations under clinical conditions. The radio-immunoassay technique[46] (now available as a commercial 'kit') is rapid, sensitive and precise but certain batches of antibody may cross-react with steroid compounds, particularly cortisol and spironolac-tone[7]. The method based on rubidium-86 uptake by red blood cells in the presence of cardiac glycosides is slower but possibly more specific. In most instances, however, the two methods give similar values[9]. Several studies have now shown that plasma digoxin con-centrations are of value in the diagnosis of digoxin toxicity[5, 8, 17, 26, 46, 47] although some overlap between toxic and non-toxic levels have been observed by most workers *(Figure 10.4)*. These investigations have shown that patients with digoxin toxicity usually have plasma concentrations of more than 2 ng/ml whilst the therapeutic range appears to be between 1 and 2 ng/ml. Assaying plasma digoxin there-fore provides the clinician with information of considerable value. Toxicity occurs in 20 per cent or more of patients treated with the drug but the diagnosis is frequently impossible to make on clinical grounds because increasing heart failure and a wide variety of both supraven-tricular and ventricular arrhythmias may be due either to overdigitaliza-tion or to the underlying condition for which the drug was being administered (underdigitalization)[18].

Since a wide range of plasma and myocardial digoxin levels is compatible with effective digitalization in different patients the therapeutic

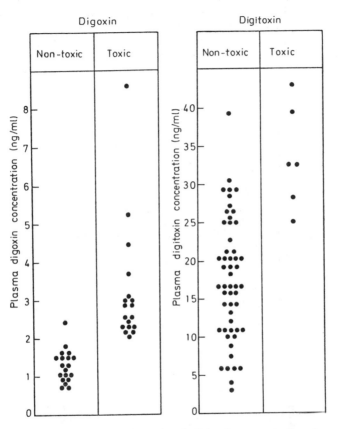

Figure 10.4. Plasma digoxin and digitoxin concentrations in non-toxic and toxic patients. Digoxin toxicity is unusual at plasma levels below 2 ng/ml and digitoxin toxicity below 25 ng/ml. (From Smith, Butler and Haber, 1969[46] and Smith and Haber, 1971[48])

concentration required by an individual patient is not readily predictable[12, 22]. In interpreting the results of plasma digoxin concentrations the time of sampling with respect to the last dose of the drug is crucial[41] (Figure 10.5).

Plasma digitoxin concentrations may also be measured by radio-immunoassay[45] using a specific antibody. Plasma levels in toxic patients are greater than those in non-toxic ones[48] (see *Figure 10.4*) but, as with digoxin, some overlap between the groups occurs. Measurements of plasma digoxin and digitoxin concentrations are therefore of considerable value in clinical practice but, as with all laboratory investigations, they must be interpreted in the light of the clinical circumstances.

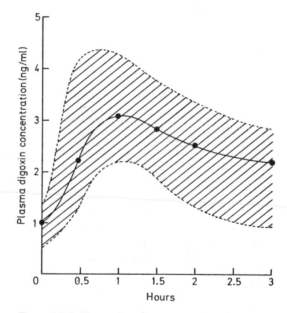

Figure 10.5. Plasma digoxin concentrations (mean and range) in 11 fully digitalized patients at various times following oral administration of 0.375 mg. (From Redfors, 1972[41])

Hydrallazine. — The relationship between dose and steady-state plasma hydrallazine concentration varies fourfold between individuals. Since the drug is largely metabolized by acetylation, which is subject to genetic polymorphism, this variability is mainly due to acetylator phenotype[54]. There appears to be an excellent relationship between steady-state plasma hydrallazine levels and hypotensive response in patients receiving concurrent therapy with propranolol. It has been suggested that estimates of plasma hydrallazine concentrations may be of value in avoiding excessive doses[54].

Practolol. — The measurement of plasma practolol concentrations appears to provide no indication of the degree of pain relief likely to be found in patients with angina pectoris[24]. This is probably because patients with severe disease tend to be non-responsive, even though given large doses which produce high plasma levels.

Anti-inflammatory drugs

Salicylates. — The first demonstration of the values of monitoring the plasma level of a drug was undertaken by Coburn[19]. He showed that 6.6 g salicylate daily in divided doses produced steady-state plasma concentrations ranging from 158 to 288 μg/ml. He observed that patients whose plasma salicylate level was more than 350 μg/ml had a prompt and progressive subsidence of both clinical and laboratory evidence of rheumatic fever; patients whose plasma concentrations were less than this showed persistent evidence of a continuing inflammatory process. Furthermore, he found that in 30 patients whose plasma salicylate was kept above 350 μg/ml none developed subsequent valvular heart disease, whilst 21 of 63 patients treated with low doses of salicylate developed this complication. Unfortunately, no detailed statistical analysis was published in this study and although numerous trials of salicylate therapy in rheumatic fever have been published subsequently, the merits of adjusting the dosage in the light of the plasma levels has never been refuted or confirmed. It has been pointed out that frequent dosage adjustments are necessary to maintain plasma salicylate concentrations between 300 and 400 μg/ml[28] — 172 alterations in 55 courses of treatment. In view of the ease with which salicylate estimations can be done, however, and of the enormous potential therapeutic benefit, monitoring of therapy in this situation is clearly advisable.

Phenylbutazone. — Phenylbutazone is used as an anti-inflammatory agent in the treatment of a variety of arthropathies, particularly rheumatoid arthritis. Burns and his colleagues[16] observed that in 60 patients treated with 800 mg daily, the steady-state concentration varied from 60 to 150 μg/ml. They also found that increasing dosage of the drug did not produce a directly comparable increase in steady-state plasma concentration. More recent studies have indicated that the incidence of side-effects during phenylbutazone therapy is much greater in patients with plasma concentrations above 90–100 μg/ml and that over-all optimal therapeutic responses can be obtained with plasma concentrations in the range of 50–80 μg/ml[49]. Further studies are needed, however, to elucidate more clearly the therapeutic and toxic levels.

143

Drugs acting on the respiratory system

Steady-state plasma concentrations of theophylline in patients receiving 200 mg 6-hourly range from 5 to 30 μg/ml[30]. This variability appears to be due to interindividual differences in the rate of metabolism. The effective therapeutic range of plasma theophylline levels for relief of bronchospasm appears to be 10–20 μg/ml[29, 30, 52], whilst toxicity usually (though not always) occurs at plasma levels above this. In a recent study it was observed that 25 per cent of asthmatic patients receiving theophylline benefited from measurements of plasma levels because of the improved dosage schedules that could be designed[30].

A pharmacokinetic approach to therapeutics clearly offers an exciting prospect for improving drug therapy in clinical practice and there are a number of therapeutic situations where this approach may be of considerable benefit. Plasma level determinations, however, cannot replace clinical observation of drug effects and must always be interpreted in the light of the prevailing clinical circumstances. They are unnecessary if the patient responds satisfactorily to a carefully chosen dosage schedule but can greatly clarify the situation when the desired therapeutic effect is not achieved or when toxic effects are suspected.

References

1. Allen, J. G., Calne, D. B., Davies, C. A. and Reid, J. L. (1971). 'Relationship of plasma concentration of levodopa to clinical response in Parkinsonism.' Br. J. Pharmac. 43, 464–465P
2. Åsberg, M., Chronholm, B., Sjöqvist, F. and Tuck, D. (1970). 'Correlation of subjective side effects with plasma concentrations of nortriptyline.' Br. med. J. 4, 18–21
3. Åsberg, M., Cronholm, B., Sjöqvist, F. and Tuck, D. (1971). 'Relationship between plasma level and therapeutic effect of nortriptyline.' Br. med. J. 3, 331–334
4. Baastrup, P. C., Poulsen, J. C., Schou, M., Thomsen, K. and Amdisen, A. (1970). 'Prophylactic lithium: double blind discontinuation in manic-depressive and recurrent-depressive disorders.' Lancet 2, 326–330
5. Beller, G. A., Smith, T. W., Abelmann, W. H., Haber, E. and Hood, W. B. (1971). 'Digitalis intoxication. A prospective clinical study with serum level correlations.' New. Engl. J. Med. 284, 989–997
6. Berlin, A., Agurell, S., Borgå, O., Lund, L. and Sjöqvist, F. (1972). 'Micromethod for the determination of diphenylhydantoin in plasma and cerebrospinal fluid – a comparison between a

gas chromatographic and a spectrophotometric method.' *Scand. J. clin. Lab. Invest.* **29**, 281–287

7. Bertler, Å. (1972). Personal communication.
8. Bertler, Å. and Redfors, A. (1970). 'Plasma levels of digoxin in relation to toxicity.' *Acta Pharmac. Toxic.* **29** (Suppl. 3), 281–287
9. Bertler, Å. and Redfors, A. (1972). 'Plasma glycoside level in relation to toxicity.' *Proc. 5th Int. Congr. Pharmacol.*, pp. 60–61. Basle: Karger
10. Bewick, M., Ogg, C. S., Parsons, V., Snowdon, S. A. and Manuel, L. (1972). 'Further assessment of rosette inhibition test on clinical organ transplantation.' *Br. med. J.* **3**, 491–494
11. Bigger, J. T., Schmidt, D. H. and Kutt, H. (1968). 'Relationship between the plasma level of diphenylhydantoin sodium and its cardiac antiarrhythmic effects.' *Circulation* **38**, 363–374
12. Binnion, P. F., Morgan, L. M., Stevenson, H. M. and Fletcher, E. (1969). 'Plasma and myocardial digoxin concentrations in patients on oral therapy.' *Br. Heart J.* **31**, 636–640
13. Borgå, O., Lund, L. and Sjöqvist, F. (1969). 'Bestämning av difenylhydantoin (DFH) i plasma hos patienter med epilepsi.' *Läkartidningen* **66**, 89–98
14. Braithwaite, R. A., Goulding, R., Theano, G., Bailey, J. and Coppen, A. (1972). 'Plasma concentration of amitriptyline and clinical response.' *Lancet* **1**, 1297–1300
15. Buchthal, F., Svensmark, O. and Schiller, P. J. (1960). 'Clinical and electroencephalographic correlations with serum levels of diphenylhydantoin.' *Archs Neurol., Chicago* **2**, 624–630
16. Burns, J. J., Rose, R. K., Chenkin, T., Goldman, A., Schulert, A. and Brodie, B. B. (1953). 'The physiological disposition of phenylbutazone (Butazolidin) in man and a method for its estimation in biological material.' *J. Pharmac. exp. Ther.* **109**, 346–357
17. Chamberlain, D. A., White, R. J., Howard, M. R. and Smith, T. W. (1970). 'Plasma digoxin concentration in patients with atrial fibrillation.' *Br. med. J.* **3**, 429–432
18. Chung, K-Y. (1968). 'Cardiac failure from digitalis intoxication.' In *Drug-induced Disease*, Vol. 3. Ed. by L. Meyler and H. M. Peck. Amsterdam: Excerpta Medica
19. Coburn, A. F. (1943). 'Salicylate therapy in rheumatic fever. A rational technique.' *Bull. Johns Hopkins Hosp.* **73**, 435–464
20. Conn, H. L. and Luchi, R. J. (1964). 'Some cellular and metabolic considerations relating to the action of quinidine as a prototype antiarrhythmic agent.' *Am. J. Med.* **37**, 685–699
21. Coppen, A., Noguera, R., Bailey, J., Burns, B. H., Swani, M. S., Hare, F. H., Gardner, R. and Maggs, R. (1971). 'Prophylactic lithium in affective disorders. Controlled trial.' *Lancet* **2**, 275–279

145

22. Evered, D. C., Chapman, C. and Hayter, C. J. (1970). 'Measurement of plasma digoxin concentration by radioimmunoassay.' *Br. med. J.* **3**, 427–428

23. Fry, D. E. and Marks, V. (1971). 'Value of plasma-lithium monitoring.' *Lancet* **1**, 886–889

24. George, C. F., Nagle, R. E. and Pentecost, B. L. (1970). 'Practolol in the treatment of angina pectoris. A double blind trial.' *Br. med. J.* **1**, 402–404

25. Gianelly, R., Groeben, J. O. von der, Spivack, A. P. and Harrison, D. C. (1967). 'Effect of lidocaine on ventricular arrhythmias in patients with coronary heart disease.' *New Engl. J. Med.* **277**, 1215–1219

26. Grahame-Smith, D. G. and Everest, M. S. (1969). 'Measurement of digoxin in plasma and its use in diagnosis of digoxin intoxication.' *Br. med. J.* **1**, 286–289

27. Hibble, A. G. and Grahame-Smith, D. G. (1972). 'The plasma digoxin concentration, red cell rubidium 86 uptake and control of ventricular rate in patients being digitalised for atrial fibrillation.' *Clin. Sci.* **42**, 3P

28. Holt, K. S. (1954). 'Salicylates in rheumatic fever. Difficulties experienced in treating children with large doses.' *Lancet* **2**, 1197–1199

29. Jackson, R. H., McHenry, J. I., Moreland, F. B., Raymer, W. J. and Etter, R. L. (1964). 'Clinical evaluation of Elixophyllin with correlation of pulmonary function studies and theophylline serum levels in acute and chronic asthmatic patients.' *Dis. Chest.* **45**, 75–85

30. Jenne, J. W., Wyze, E., Rood, F. S. and Macdonald, F. M. (1972). 'Pharmacokinetics of theophylline. Application to adjustment of the clinical use of aminophylline.' *Clin. Pharmac. Ther.* **13**, 349–360

31. Koch-Weser, J. (1971). 'Pharmacokinetics of procainamide in man.' *Ann. N.Y. Acad. Sci.* **179**, 370–382

32. Koch-Weser, J. (1972). 'Correlation of plasma levels of antiarrhythmic drugs with their pharmacologic effects.' *Proc. 5th Int. Congr. Pharmacol.*, 56. Basle: Karger

33. Koch-Weser, J., Klein, S. W., Foo-Cantu, L. L., Kastor, J. A. and Desanctis, R. W. (1969). 'Antiarrhythmic prophylaxis with procainamide in acute myocardial infarction.' *New Engl. J. Med.* **281**, 1253–1260

34. Kutt, H. and McDowell, F. (1968). 'Management of epilepsy with diphenylhydantoin sodium.' *J. Am. med. Ass.* **203**, 969–972

35. Kutt, H., Winters, W., Kokenge, R. and McDowell, F. (1964). 'Diphenylhydantoin metabolism, blood levels, and toxicity.' *Archs Neurol., Chicago* **11**, 642–648

36. Lund, L., Lunde, P. K., Rane, A., Borgå, O. and Sjöqvist, F. (1971). 'Plasma protein binding, plasma concentrations, and

effects of diphenylhydantoin in man.' *Ann. N.Y. Acad. Sci.* **179**, 723–728

37. Lunde, P. K. M., Rane, A., Yaffe, S. J., Lund, L. and Sjöqvist, F. (1970). 'Plasma protein binding of diphenylhydantoin in man: interaction with other drugs and the effect of temperature and plasma dilution.' *Clin. Pharmac. Ther.* **11**, 846–855

38. Munro, A., Bewick, M., Manuel, L., Cameron, J. S., Ellis, F. G., Boulton-Jones, M. and Ogg, C. S. (1971). 'Clinical evaluation of a Rosette inhibition test in renal allotransplantation.' *Br. med. J.* **3**, 271–276

39. O'Reilly, R. A. and Aggeler, P. M. (1970). 'Determinants of the response to oral anticoagulant drugs in man.' *Pharmac. Rev.* **22**, 35–96

40. Rane, A., Lunde, P. K. M., Jalling, B., Yaffe, S. J. and Sjöqvist, F. (1971). 'Plasma protein binding of diphenylhydantoin in normal and hyperbilirubinemic infants.' *J. Pediat.* **78**, 877–882

41. Redfors, A. (1972). 'Plasma digoxin concentration – its relation to digoxin dosage and clinical effects in patients with atrial fibrillation.' *Br. Heart J.* **34**, 383–391

42. Reidenberg, M. M., Odar-Cederloff, I., von Bahr, C., Borgå, O. and Sjöqvist, F. (1971). 'Protein binding of diphenylhydantoin and desmethylimipramine in plasma from patients with poor renal function.' *New Engl. J. Med.* **285**, 264–267

43. Sedvall, G., Pettersson, U. and Fyrö, B. (1970). 'Individual differences in serum levels of lithium in human subjects receiving fixed doses of lithium carbonate. Relation to renal lithium clearance and body weight.' *Pharmacologia Clin.* **2**, 231–235

44. Sjöqvist, F., Hammer, W., Ideström, C-M., Lind, M., Tuck, D. and Åsberg, M. (1968). 'Plasma level of monomethylated tricyclic antidepressants and side-effects in man.' In *Toxicity and Side-Effects of Psychotropic Drugs,* Excerpta Medica Int. Congr. Series, **145**, 246–257

45. Smith, T. W. (1970). 'Radioimmunoassay for serum digitoxin concentration: methodology and clinical experience.' *J. Pharmac. exp. Ther.* **175**, 352–360

46. Smith, T. W., Butler, V. P. and Haber, E. (1969). 'Determination of therapeutic and toxic serum digoxin concentrations by radioimmunoassay.' *New Engl. J. Med.* **281**, 1212–1216

47. Smith, T. W. and Haber, E. (1970). 'Digoxin intoxication: the relationship of clinical presentation to serum digoxin concentration.' *J. clin. Invest.* **49**, 2377–2386

48. Smith, T. W. and Haber, E. (1971). 'The clinical value of serum digitalis glycoside concentrations in the evaluation of drug toxicity.' *Ann. N.Y. Acad. Sci.* **179**, 322–337

49. Strandberg, B. (1964). 'Phenylbutazone in the treatment of rheumatic disorders. A survey and clinical report.' *Acta rheum. scand.* Suppl. 10, 1–50

50. Svensmark, O. and Buchthal. F. (1964). 'Diphenylhydantoin and phenobarbital.' *Am. J. Dis. Child.* **108**, 82–87
51. Thomson, P. D., Rowland, M. and Melmon, K. C. (1971). 'The influence of heart failure, liver disease and renal failure on the disposition of lidocaine in man.' *Am. Heart J.* **82**, 417–421
52. Turner-Warrick, M. (1957). 'Study of theophylline plasma levels after oral administration of new theophylline compounds.' *Br. med. J.* **2**, 67–69
53. Walter, C. J. S. (1971). 'Clinical significance of plasma imipramine levels.' *Proc. R. Soc. Med.* **64**, 282–285
54. Zacest, R. and Koch-Weser, J. (1972). 'Relation to hydralazine plasma concentration to dosage and hypotensive action.' *Clin. Pharmac. Ther.* **13**, 420–425

Calculation of Drug Dosage in Renal Failure on the Basis of Creatinine Clearance

The method of calculating dosage in renal failure is based on the linear relationship which exists between the elimination rate constant and glomerular filtration rate (as assessed by creatinine clearance)[1] for drugs which are excreted partially or completely by the kidney (see Chapter 8).

The following must be determined.

(1)   Maintenance dose of the drug (M) and the dosage interval (T) which would have been used had the patient had normal renal function.

(2)   The patient's creatinine clearance.

(3)   The patient's elimination rate constant for the drug ($k_{patient}$). This can be determined graphically by use of the chart shown in *Figure A.1.*

The normal elimination rate constant for the drug (k_{normal}) is found by reference to Table A.1 and is marked on the chart on the right-hand ordinate (corresponding to a creatinine clearance of 120 ml/min) — for ampicillin this is 0.6 hours^{-1}. The elimination rate constant when creatinine clearance is zero ($k_{anephric}$) is similarly marked on the left-hand ordinate — for ampicillin this is 0.11 hours^{-1} — and a line is drawn between these two points. The patient's elimination rate constant can be interpolated.

The dosage schedule is calculated as follows.

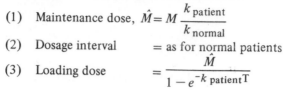

(1) Maintenance dose, $\hat{M} = M \dfrac{k_{\text{patient}}}{k_{\text{normal}}}$

(2) Dosage interval = as for normal patients

(3) Loading dose $= \dfrac{\hat{M}}{1 - e^{-k_{\text{patient}}T}}$

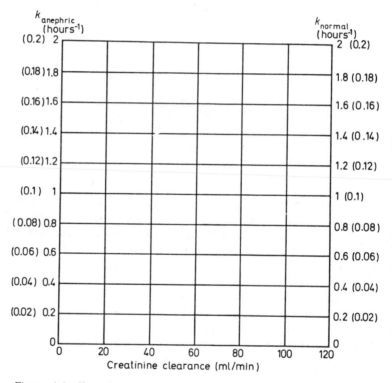

Figure A.1. Chart for the graphical determination of individual elimination constants ($k_{patient}$) *in patients with impaired renal function. See text for use: e.g. ampicillin* ($k_{anephric} = 0.11$; $k_{normal} = 0.60$) *for patient with creatinine clearance 40 ml/min, $k_{patient} = 0.27$. (From Dettli, Spring and Ryter, 1971[1])*

Calculation of the loading dose, though complicated in appearance, is simple to perform with the use of *natural exponential function* tables (e.g. Documenta Geigy). The use of a loading dose in patients with poor renal function is essential if steady-state plasma levels are to be reached quickly.

TABLE A.1. Elimination Rate Constants (hours^{-1}) for Various Drugs in Normal and Anephric Patients

Drug	$k_{anephric}$ (hours^{-1})	k_{normal} (hours^{-1})
Ampicillin	0.11	0.6
Benzylpenicillin	0.03	1.4
Carbenicillin	0.04	0.45
Cephalexin	0.03	0.7
Cephaloridine	0.03	0.4
Cephalothin	0.06	1.4
Chloramphenicol	0.2	0.3
Colistin	0.08	0.31
Digitoxin	0.003	0.004
Digoxin	0.008	0.017
Doxycycline	0.03	0.03
Erythromycin	0.13	0.5
Gentamicin	0.02	0.3
Kanamycin	0.01	0.25
Lincomycin	0.06	0.15
Methicillin	0.17	1.4
Oxacillin	0.35	1.4
Polymyxin B	0.02	0.16
Rifampicin	0.25	0.25
Streptomycin	0.01	0.27
Sulphamethoxazole	0.07	0.07
Trimethoprim	0.03	0.07
Vancomycin	0.003	0.12

From Dettli, Spring and Ryter (1971)[1].

If a drug is to be given by continuous intravenous infusion, the maintenance dose is calculated as above. Again, a loading dose should be given. It is calculated as follows.

(3a)   Loading dose (infusion) $= \dfrac{\hat{M}}{T \cdot k_{patient}}$

For reasons outlined in Chapter 8, the dosage schedule calculated in this manner does not obviate the necessity of measuring the plasma drug concentrations whenever possible. Appropriate dose adjustments should be made if indicated.

Reference

1.   Dettli, L., Spring, P. and Ryter, S. (1971). 'Multiple dose kinetics and drug dosage in patients with kidney disease.' *Acta Pharmac. Tox.* **29** (Suppl. 3), 211–224

APPENDIX B

Antibiotic Dosage in Renal Failure

The loading dose of antibiotic given in renal failure [1] is the same as that in patients with normal renal function. Maintenance doses of half the loading dose are given at intervals as shown in Table B.1. The drugs have been subdivided into four groups:

Group   I: major dosage reduction (serum concentrations should be monitored)
    II: minor dosage reduction
    III: no dosage reduction
    IV: to be avoided altogether

TABLE B.1

Maintenance doses

Group	Drug	Maintenance dose intervals in renal impairment	
		Moderate (plasma creatinine 3–8 mg%)	Severe (plasma creatinine >8 mg%)
I	Colistin	1–2 days	2–3 days
	Gentamicin	1 day	2 days
	Kanamycin	1–2 days	3–4 days
	Streptomycin	1–2 days	5 days
	Vancomycin	3–5 days	7–14 days
II	Benzylpenicillin*	6 hours	8 hours
	Carbenicillin*	6 hours	8 hours
	Cephalothin	6 hours	8 hours
	Co-trimoxazole	12 hours	1 day
III	Ampicillin		
	Cloxacillin		
	Erythromycin		
	Fucidin		
	Isoniazid		
	Lincomycin		
	Novobiocin		
	Rifampicin		
IV	Cephaloridine		
	Chloramphenicol		
	Nitrofurantoin		
	Tetracyclines		

*For high dose penicillin therapy, greater dosage restriction is required and serum concentrations should be monitored.

Reference

1. Jones, N. F. and Wing, A.J. (1971). 'Renal disease.' In *A Guide to the Therapy of Common Diseases*, pp. 25–54. Ed. by W. I. Cranston. Lancaster: Medical and Technical Publ.

APPENDIX C

Some Physical Properties and Pharmacokinetic Parameters of Drugs in Common Use

The table below is incomplete. The reader is invited to fill in the missing data.
Abbreviations: A = acid, B = base, B₄ = base with quaternary ammonium group, Alc. = alcohol, Glyc. = glycoside, S = steroid.

I Drug	II Nature	III pK_a	IV Percentage protein bound	V Elimination T½ (hours)	VI Percentage excreted unchanged (following parenteral administration)
Acetaminophen	Alc.	–	25	2	1–3
Acetazolamide	A	7.2	90–95	2.4–5.8	100
Acetohexamide	A			5–8	<2

	Type	pKa				Notes
Acetophenetidin	Subst. amide	—	30	1	<1	
Actinomycin D	Chromopeptide				10	
Allopurinol	B	9.4	0	2–8	<10	
Amantadine	B				90	
Amiloride	B	8.7			100	
Aminocaproic acid	Ampholyte	4.4, 10.7			>95	
Aminopyrine	B	5.0	15–20	2–7	3	
Aminosalicylic acid	A	3.2	58–73	0.75	40	
Amitriptyline	B	9.4	96			
Amphetamine	B	9.8		10–30*	70–90*	*urinary pH-dependent
Amphotericin B	Ampholyte	5.5, 10.0		24	5–40	
Ampicillin	A	2.5, 7.2	25	2	50	
Amylobarbitone	A	7.7	61	20	<1	
Antipyrine	B	1.4	0–8	6–24	0–5	
Apomorphine	B	7.2, 8.9			25	
Atropine	B	9.8	50	13–38	25	
Aspirin	A	3.5		0.25	<1	hydrolysed to salicylic acid
Barbitone	A	7.8	0–17		90	
Benzylpenicillin	A	2.8	46–58	0.25–0.5	58–90	
Betahistine	B	3.5, 9.7		<2	—	*dose-dependent
Bishydroxycoumarin	A	5.7	95–99	7–74*		

– continued overleaf

155

Drug	Nature	pK_a	Percentage bound	$T_{1/2}$	Percentage excreted unchanged
Bupivacaine	B	8.1	95	2.5	<5
Burimamide	B	7.5	5	2	>50
Butobarbitone	A	7.9	26		
Caffeine	B	0.8			10
Capreomycin	Peptide*			3	70
Carbamazepine	Amide		72	25–59	
Carbenicillin	A	2.6, 2.7	47	1–2	80
Carbenoxolone			>99		<1
Cephalexin	A	5.2, 7.3	15–30	0.5–1	>90
Cephaloridine	A		<5	1.5	70
Cephalothin	A	2.5	56	0.5–1	60–90
Chlorambucil	B	8.0			
Chloramphenicol	Alc.	–	25	1.6–3.3	5–15
Chlordiazepoxide	B	4.6		8–28	5–15
Chlormethiazole	B	3.2	0	1	0
Chloroquine	B	8.4, 10.8	55	120	10–24
Chlorpheniramine	B	9.2	70	1–1.5	13–30
Chlorpromazine	B	9.3	91–99	2–31	1–6
Chlorpropamide	A	4.8	80	24–42	10–30
Chlortetracycline	B	3.3, 7.4, 9.3	47	5.6	20
Clindamycin	B	6.9	67–93	2–4	5–15

*4 different compounds

Clofibrate	A		98	12	3–24
Clonidine	B			20	41–47
Cloxacillin	A	2.7	95	1.5	35
Codeine	B	6.0		1.6–5.0	40–80
Colistin	B		10	0.5	
Cortisol	S				
Cyclizine	B	8.2			
Cyclobarbitone	A	7.3	70	3–6.5	35–40
Cyclophosphamide	B			0.4–3.5	8–10
Cytarabine	B	4.3			10
Dactinomycin		Chromopeptide			
Dapsone	A	1.2–2.5	72–80	17–21	
Daunorubicin	A			6–63	15–30
Demethylchlor-tetracycline	B	7.2, 9.4	41	12	42
Desipramine	B	9.5	73–92	12–54	<5
Dexamethazone	S			3.5	
Dextromoramide	B	7.0		1.5–5	
Dextropropoxyphene	B	6.3			25
Diamorphine	B	7.6			<1
Diazepam	B	3.3	96	48–144	<5
Diazoxide	A		99	26	<0.5
Dicoumarol	A	5.7	95–99	7–74*	

*dose-dependent

– continued overleaf

Drug	Nature	pK_a	Percentage bound	$T_{1/2}$	Percentage excreted unchanged	
Digitoxin	Glyc.	—	95	100–200	30	
Digoxin	Glyc.	—	23	30–40	85	
Dihydrocodeine	B	8.8	7.9	6		
Diphenhydramine	B	8.3		2.5		
Diphenoxylate	B				0	
Diphenylhydantoin	A	8.3	87	10–42*	<1	*dose-dependent
Disodium cromoglycate	A	2.0	69	1	100*	*of drug absorbed
Doxycycline	Ampholyte	3.4, 7.7, 9.7	93	20–24	45	
Droperidol	B	7.6				
Emepronium	B				70	
Emetine	B	5.8, 6.6		2		
Ephedrine	B	9.6				
Ergometrine	B	7.3				
Ergonovine	B	7.3				
Erythromycin	B	8.8	18	1.4	15	
Eserine	B	8.5				
Ethacrynic acid	A	3.5		0.5–1	20	
Ethambutol	B	6.5, 9.0	8	4	80	
Ethionamide	B		10	2.2	2–8	
Ethosuximide	A	9.3	–	60*	20	*$T_{1/2}$ 30 hours in children
Ethyl biscoumacetate	A	3.1	90	2–3.5		

Fenfluramine	B	9.9	32	14–30	2–12	
Flucloxacillin	A	2.7	95	2.5	60	
Fludrocortisone	S	–	70–79	0.5	10–20	
5-Fluorouracil	B	8.1		<1	100	
Frusemide	A	3.7	75	1.2	86–100	
Gentamicin	B	*	25–30	2.3	0	*4 different compounds
Glibenclamide	A			5–7	<1	
Glutethimide	Ampholyte		54	5.1–22	25–50	
Griseofulvin					50	
Guanethidine	B		0	1–2.5*	<1	*dose-dependent
Heparin	A				<5	
Heroin	B	7.6		6		
Hexobarbitone	A	8.2				
Homatropine	B	9.7				
Hydrallazine	B			2–6*		*dose-dependent
Hydrochlorothiazide	A	7.9, 9.2				
Hyoscine	B	8.1			69–77	
Hyoscine N-butylbromide	B_4	–	10			
Ibuprofen	A	4.4		7.6	<2	
Imipramine	B	9.5	75–96	1.5	<1	
Indomethacin	A		90	1.8	0	
Indoramine	B	7.7				

– continued overleaf

Drug	Nature	pK_a	Percentage bound	$T_{1/2}$	Percentage excreted unchanged
Iprindole	B	8.2			5
Isocarboxazid	B				2
Isoniazid	B		0	0.8–5	4–27
Isoprenaline	B	8.6			
Isoxsuprine	B	8.0, 9.8		1.25	0
Kanamycin	B		10	3–5	52–90
Levallorphan	B	45			
Levodopa	Amino acid	2.3, 8.7, 9.9		2.5	<1
Lignocaine	B	7.9	70	1–2	<5
Lincomycin	B	7.6	80–90	4.4–4.7	10–15
Lithium	—		0	24	100
Lorazepam	Ampholyte	1.3, 11.5		10–24	0
Lysergide	B	3.3, 7.8		1.7	
Mecamylamine	B	11.2			
Mefenamic acid	A	4.2	98.5		
Melphalan	B		50–60		
Mepacrine	B	7.7, 10.3	90	120	4
Meperidine	B	8.7	40	5.5	5
Mephenesin	Glycerol ether				<2
Meprobamate	—	—		7–17	8–19
Metaraminol	B	8.6			

					*pH-dependent
Methadone	B	8.6	40	10–47	5–22*
Methicillin	A	2.8	37–50	0.5–1.75	25–82
Methohexitone	A	7.9, 8.3	73		<1
Methotrexate	A	4.8, 5.5	40–50	1.5	85–100
Methotrimeprazine	B	9.2		1	1–2
Methoxamine	B	4.8			
Methylamphetamine	B	10.0			
Methyldopa	Amino acid		<20	2.0	20–55
Metoclopramide					24
Metronidazole				6	60–70
Morphine	B	7.9, 8.1, 9.9		10–44	1
Nalidixic acid	A	6.7	80	1.1–2	2–6
Nalorphine	B	7.8			<4
Nitrazepam	B	3.2, 10.8	85	18–28	36
Nitrofurantoin	A	7.2	70	0.3	5
Nortriptyline	B		94	15–90	2–3
Novobiocin		4.3, 9.1	96	2.3	2
Orciprenaline	B	8.9, 11.8		1.5	2
Orphenadrine	B	8.4	20	10	<2
Oxacillin	A		94	0.5	30
Oxazepam	Ampholyte	1.7, 11.6		7–14	0
Oxyphenbutazone	A	4.7	90	27–64	<5
Oxytetracycline	B	3.3, 7.3, 9.1	20–35	9.6	70

– continued overleaf

162

Drug	Nature	pK_a	Percentage bound	$T_{1/2}$	Percentage excreted unchanged
Papaverine	B	6.4			
Paracetamol	Alc.	–	25	2	1–3
Penicillamine	B	1.8, 7.9, 10.5			
Pentaerythritol tetranitrate				7.1	0
Pentazocine	B			2	2–5
Pentobarbitone	A	8.1	40–65	21–39	20
Pentolinium	B_4				100
Perphenazine	B	7.8			
Pethidine	B	8.7	40	5.5	5
Phenacetin	Subst. amide	–	30	1	<1
Phenindione	A			6	
Phenobarbitone	A	7.2	40	53–140	11–25
Phenoxybenzamine	B				1
Phenoxymethyl-penicillin	A	2.7			
Phentolamine	B				10
Phenylbutazone	A	4.5	90–98	52–120*	1 *dose-dependent
Phenytoin	A	8.3	87	10–42*	<1 *dose-dependent
Physostigmine	B	8.5			
Piperazine	B	5.7, 9.8			

Polymyxin B			10	6	60–90
Practolol	B	9.5	<10	6–12	85–100
Prednisolone	S	–	90	2.5–3	0
Prenylamine	B		>95	6	<1
Prilocaine	B	7.9	50		
Primidone	A			3.3–12.5	
Probenecid	A	3.4	75–94	4–12	1–5
Procaine	B	8.8			
Procainamide	B	9.2	15	2.5–4.7	40–54
Prochlorperazine	B	8.1	0		
Promazine	B	9.4			
Promethazine	B	9.1	7.5		
Propantheline	B				50
Propranolol	B	9.45	>90	2.3	
Protriptyline	B		92		
Pyrazinamide	B	0.5			
Pyridostigmine	B$_4$				2–16
Pyrimethamine	B	7.2		96	
Quinacrine	B	7.7, 10.3	90	120	4
Quinalbarbitone	A	7.9	65–75		10
Quinidine	B	4.3, 8.4	60–80	2	10–50
Quinine	B	4.3, 8.4	75–90		
Reserpine	B	6.1			

– continued overleaf

Drug	Nature	pK_a	Percentage bound	$T_{1/2}$	Percentage excreted unchanged
Rifampicin	Ampholyte		85	1.5–5	15
Salbutamol	B	9.3, 10.3		2–4	40–50
Salicylazosulpha-pyridine	A	0.6, 2.4, 9.7, 11.8		4.6–9.8	2–10
Salicylic acid	A	3.0	75	6–8*	*dose-dependent
Secobarbital	A	7.9	65–75		10
Streptomycin	B		34	2.4–2.7	30–80
Succinylcholine	B_4			0.03	0
Succinylsulphathiazole	A	4.5			
Sulphadiazine	A	6.3	20–68	15–17	43–85
Sulphadimethoxine	A	6.3	90–99	20–40	<5
Sulphadimidine	A		55		
Sulphafurazole	A	4.9	75–95	4–7	50–70
Sulphamethizole	A	5.4	90		
Sulphamethoxazole	A	6.0	60–70	8–12	10–30
Sulphamethoxy-pyridazine	A	6.7	80	24	30–60
Sulphasalazine	A	0.6, 2.4, 9.7, 11.8		4.6–9.8	2–10
Sulphathiazole	A	7.1	55–80	4–11	54–77
Sulphinpyrazone	A	2.8	95	3	25–50

Sulthiame	A				30
Suxamethonium	B$_4$			0.03	0
Terbutaline	B	10.1	25	3.5–4	7–8
Tetracycline	B	3.3, 7.8, 9.7	25–75	8.5	60
Theophylline	B	0.7	15	3–9.5	10
Thiopentone	A	7.6	75	4	<1
Thyroxine			>99	80–180	<5
Tolazoline	B	10.3	23		
Tolbutamide	A	5.4	97	4–9	
Tranexamic acid	Ampholyte	4.3, 10.6		2	>95
Trifluoperazine	B	8.1	>99		
Tri-iodothyronine				35–60	<5
Trimethoprim	B	6.4	30–60	8–12	40–70
Trimipramine	B		94		
Tubocurarine	B$_4$				33
Vancomycin	B		10	6	30–100
Vinblastine	B	5.4, 7.4			<5
Vincristine	B	5.0, 7.4		1.5	<5
Warfarin	A		97	15–58	

Index